The Modern Woman's Guide to

CHOOSING A PLASTIC SURGEON

Breast, Body, Buttocks

by William Bruno, MD

The Modern Woman's Guide to

Choosing a Plastic Surgeon
Breast, Body, Buttocks

Proudly printed in the USA

Table of Contents

Introduction 6

Chapter 1: Being Your Best "You" 10

Chapter 2: Is Plastic Surgery Right for You? 20

Chapter 3: Mirror, Mirror…Selecting a Procedure 28

Chapter 4: Choosing the Right Surgeon 76

Chapter 5: Go for It! 95

About the Author... 103

Patient Reviews 108

The photos displayed in this book are
actual patients of Dr. William Bruno.

I would like to dedicate this book to my parents,
Lucille and Fred, and to all those patients who
trusted me as their surgeon.

Introduction

Nip/Tuck. Botched. The Swan. Doctor 90210. Extreme Makeover. Despite the explosion of reality-based TV shows about plastic surgery, there is still no easy way to obtain unbiased, medically accurate information about plastic surgery. Each show has its own agenda, its producers their own views on the subject. Each website you Google may or may not contain medically accurate information, and they, too, have their own biases. Newspaper and magazine articles are more often than not simply advertisements in disguise. Doctors' offices pump out press releases with specific story "hooks" — hoping to get a pick-up in the media. The media, for its own part, has airtime and space to fill — their twenty-four-hour-a-day, seven-day-a-week broadcasts have voracious appetites that are never satisfied. So where can you, as a non-medical professional, go to learn what is real about plastic surgery and which physicians are reputable, and even more importantly, which ones are not?

That has been my simple goal in writing this book — helping you to distinguish hype from reality and giving you the confidence to move forward to the next step, whatever that might be — scheduling an initial consultation, or perhaps realizing that you're not ready for plastic surgery just yet after all. Whatever your goals are, it is my sincere hope that this book will prove to be a valuable introduction to the sometimes confusing world of plastic surgery. It will empower you with easy-to-understand knowledge and action steps. You might wish to pour over every section, reading each in succession. Or you might decide to skip straight to the section that most interests you. Either way, it's my hope that this book can be your trusted resource.

My story

At the age of five, I decided that I was going to become a doctor. I know it's unusual for most people to be able to choose their life path at such a young age, but for me, it wasn't so much that I chose medicine — but rather that *it* chose me.

When I was four years old, I was diagnosed with a genetic disease called juvenile rheumatoid arthritis. This condition affected my knee joints primarily, causing them to swell up tremendously, and I remember the pain at night from just the weight of the sheets on my knees. Walking, as you can imagine, was difficult — and I became somewhat of a permanent fixture at my doctors' offices, having to get my knees aspirated on a regular basis. We were living in New Jersey at the time, and it wasn't long after I was diagnosed that I was sent to Boston to seek specialist care. Unlike most kids in my situation, I didn't resent having to go see so many doctors — actually I enjoyed it. I liked watching them at work — taking my vital signs, etc., and it was clear that some of them genuinely cared about me and were doing everything they could to help me get better, which left a real impression on me. My family and I made the trip to Boston regularly, until I was six years old, which is when (thankfully) I made a full recovery and went on to play Little League baseball and all the sports I loved so much, that until then I'd only been able to watch from the sidelines.

Fast forward to medical school. I studied at Hahnemann University School of Medicine in Pennsylvania, did a surgical internship at Stanford University and completed my general surgery residency at St. Louis University Medical Center. I went on to do a sub-specialization in microsurgery at Eastern Virginia Medical Center. I was growing more and more interested in the advancements being made in plastic surgery during my plastic surgery fellowship at Duke University, which combined my love of medicine and artistry into one. As a child I used to paint and draw a lot, especially dinosaurs and cartoons, but like many kids I shelved my creative talents when I went to high school, in favor of doing sports and focusing on my "serious" studies.

Plastic surgery really is artistry in medicine. I love that I'm treating both men and women of all ages, and working on all parts of the human body, instead of just one specialized anatomic area. The subtitle of the book reads "Breast, Body, Buttocks" as these areas represent the majority of the procedures I perform; although I will also cover multiple facial procedures as well.

With over ten years of experience in plastic surgery, I can say with confidence that the only thing constant about this specialty is that it's an ever-changing science.

As a prospective patient, this book can give you the

information you need to ask a doctor the appropriate questions and begin to start understanding this complex field. It is not meant to provide specific medical advice, and *please do not* use it as your sole source of information — speak to multiple plastic surgeons when weighing your options, to find the best doctor for *you*.

Wherever you are on your journey of discovery into plastic surgery, I hope this book proves to be a valuable resource.

William Bruno, MD

William Bruno, MD
Beverly Hills, California

Chapter 1: Being Your Best "You"

"Beauty is an attitude. There's no secret."
– Estée Lauder

You've always done everything possible to look your best: hairstyle, makeup, skin, teeth, nails, healthy diet and exercise. Usually you've been pleased with the results. But maybe something's changed, and you don't *feel* you look your absolute best anymore.

Maybe it's the lines around your eyes, the way the eyelids are starting to sag at the corners. Maybe it's the way time and gravity have changed your silhouette: your breasts sag a bit more every year, or your stomach or buttocks make you self-conscious in a swimsuit. These things aren't major issues in and of themselves, of course, but you can't help thinking that you'd look better — and feel better — if *just that one thing* were adjusted, brought more into line with the fabulous rest of you.

Feeling good and looking good are two sides of the same coin. When your outer image of yourself matches the inside, you're happier, more confident and have a more positive outlook. And your inner state of mind, in turn, is reflected in your outward appearance. We exercise, eat nutritionally balanced meals, invest a good deal of time and money in our grooming, and select clothes that flatter our bodies. But even the best grooming and skin care can only do so much to slow down the aging process.

Fortunately, we live in a time where it's increasingly possible to reverse it.

"Getting work done" — cosmetic surgery or plastic surgery?

People commonly ask if there is a difference between a "plastic surgeon" and a "cosmetic surgeon". These terms may sound equal, but they're not. Plastic surgeons undergo far more extensive, detailed training than purely cosmetic surgeons, and are held to more rigorous standards of certification. The specialty of plastic surgery has a recognized national board, whereas cosmetic surgery does not. We'll go into more detail about the difference in Chapter 4, but for now it may be helpful to get a quick overview of the history of plastic surgery.

> **Doctor's Note:**
> *All board-certified plastic surgeons are trained in treating the whole body, both reconstructive and aesthetic procedures. Some plastic surgeons "specialize" more on aesthetic procedures while some perform more reconstructive procedures in their practices.*

You might think of plastic surgery as a recent development, a Hollywood-era fad that has gradually spread to the mainstream. But in fact, for thousands (yes, *thousands*) of years, people have been experimenting with altering their bodies in the name of beauty. The earliest records of reconstructive surgery are from ancient Egypt and India, when doctors developed techniques to rebuild ears and noses damaged by injury or disease. Western doctors began traveling to India in the 1700s to study surgical techniques like rhinoplasty, leading to a new subfield of "aesthetic" surgery.

By the late nineteenth century, plastic surgeons in the U.S. were reporting prominent ears, double chins and "nearly all undesirable distortions of the nose (the Roman nose, the Jewish nose) can be improved or entirely corrected by cosmetic operation." In 1901, "a noble lady" in Germany underwent the first recorded facelift in human history. Six years later, Charles C. Miller wrote a book titled Plastic Surgery: The Correction of Featural Imperfections, in which he also described procedures such as injecting paraffin (wax) into sagging or wrinkled skin. Which no one does anymore, because it had poor results.

Not every reconstructive surgeon was (or is) also a cosmetic surgeon, however. The growing divide between the respected medical community and the "beauty surgeons" (who may or may not have gone to medical school) resulted in the establishment of the American Society of Plastic Surgeons, in 1931. True plastic surgeons might also perform aesthetic operations, but the "beauty doctors" never did anything but cosmetic procedures… some with better results than others. Together with the rise of Hollywood glamour and the Miss America pageant, there was suddenly a new demand for surgeries that might not be strictly *medically* necessary, but which could significantly improve people's quality of life and career prospects.

Then, as now, the demand for plastic surgery resulted in some practitioners who had absolutely no business practicing. Geoffrey C. Gurtner puts it best in *Plastic Surgery: Principles:*

> The importance given to personal appearance produced... a horde of quacks, charlatans, and beauty doctors often working in beauty salons, exclusively on a commercial basis. They advertised in newspapers, women's magazines and yellow pages [the pre-internet Google]. They appealed to popular imagination by promising a more attractive look with simple, fast procedures on an outpatient basis, at relatively high cost and by insisting beautiful faces and noses were crucial in creating a favorable first impression for finding a job, or expanding social relationships.

The more things change, the more they stay the same. Living in the twenty-first century means you have your choice of an incredible range of treatments and procedures to preserve and enhance your natural beauty, from quick laser treatments to full body lifts. But, like any rapidly changing field, the world of plastic surgery can be daunting and confusing. There are scores of practitioners making contradictory claims. Add in the horror stories of people who've been injured or disfigured, and it's easy to become discouraged.

That's why research is so essential. Consider this book a first step to empowering yourself with knowledge. The information here is not exhaustive, and is not intended as medical advice. But it can help you — a smart woman who knows what she wants — make informed choices. The goal is to discover what procedures may be right for you, and to find the best plastic surgeon to perform them. If you educate yourself and proceed with caution, you'll be well on the way to shaping the best possible version of yourself.

"Did she or didn't she?"

No one judges you for having your teeth fixed or getting an unsightly mole removed. But say "plastic surgery," and unfortunately, society is right there to jump in with labels and judgments. So maybe you don't want anyone to know you've had (or are considering) plastic surgery. You can, of course, simply maintain plausible deniability. But consider a few other things as well: you're probably going to need time off from work, and you're definitely going to need some recovery time (not to mention a ride home after the procedure). Consider whether it will make your life easier to entrust a few people with your secret, so they can lend a helping hand. You may be surprised at how supportive people are of your goals; they may even be able to recommend a surgeon or offer helpful advice.

Here's another thing to consider: when your grandmother (or perhaps great-grandmother) was young, hair dye was taboo. That doesn't mean women didn't dye their hair — they absolutely did, and so did men — they just didn't admit it.

Hair dye was only for movie stars or "fast" women, and no respectable middle-class woman would be open about the fact that she colored her hair. It wasn't *shameful*, exactly, but it was simply not in good taste.

In fact, the ad campaign slogan for Clairol, the very first commercially marketed hair color, was: "Does she or doesn't she? Only her hairdresser knows for sure." Far from the stereotype of glamorous movie stars or *femmes fatales*, "Clairol girls" were always presented as the wholesome, next-door type. The idea was that it was supposed to be a mystery that you would transition from your natural hair color to a chemically assisted one so subtly that no one would notice. To paraphrase author Malcolm Gladwell, women thought the decision about whether or not they could be blondes, brunettes or redheads was rightfully theirs… and no one else's.

The new social attitudes that came with the commercial sale of hair color are now being echoed for plastic surgery. The only difference is that by now, women are accustomed to rewriting the rules. Today, of course, hair color is as common as makeup (also once thought to be used only by tramps, and now a regular part of the professional woman's daily regimen). Women not only admit that they dye their hair, they celebrate it. Women (and some men) choose crazy colors not found in nature, or simply rotate shades according to the seasons or our social calendars. No one thinks twice about a woman getting a haircut, color or makeup consultation before going to a big event, or for the holidays, or simply for no reason other than that she wants to. It's her right, her way of taking pride in who she is and maintaining the presentation of herself that makes her feel best. *Of course* we see it as positive and empowering; we don't have to risk the same social judgment our grandmothers did.

Is this a good comparison with plastic surgery? Well, yes and no. Certainly the art and science of cosmetic procedures has come a long way from those humble nose-repairing origins. Of course you don't (and shouldn't!) change your body as frequently as you change your hair color or style. And definitely don't feel that you have to experiment beyond the bounds of what you're comfortable with; unlike hair and makeup, surgery is relatively permanent. But thinking of plastic surgery as something to be less-than-proud of is an older way of thinking, one not in keeping with the twenty-first century narrative of acceptance and empowerment. Your body is your own business, and you have every right to make decisions about it. Whether you choose to share those decisions widely, with only a few, or with no one at all is up to you.

That being said, there's a reason that much of the best plastic surgery is hard to detect. Remember, less is more. Others may not consciously notice the specific changes you've made, but they'll see that something is somehow different about you. You want the kind of results that people don't notice too much, rather than the kind of dramatic overhaul that we've all seen pictures of in the media. There are even proactive treatments, such as Botox, to prevent wrinkles before they occur. The risks now are fewer, the results better and the recovery times shorter than ever before.

Before you make a decision, you'll need to carefully consider what type of plastic surgery may be right for you — or whether it's what you're really looking for at all. Chapter 2 covers some helpful information about the process of educating yourself and preparing mentally for this important step in your life.

Of course you'll need to know about the different types of surgeries that are available, along with their benefits and potential drawbacks. Chapter 3 is entirely devoted to explaining the most common cosmetic procedures, as well as some you may not be as familiar with (but which might just make you think, "Yes, that's the one for me!") In this chapter I've also included, consultation-style, some of the questions I've heard from patients and prospective patients, along with my answers to their questions, to give you an even more in-depth understanding of these procedures, and hopefully also to spark your own thoughts about the questions you in particular may find you have. [It is important to note, however, that these questions and answers, as with the rest of this book, should in no way be understood as exhaustive, or as a substitute for an actual consultation with your own physician. This book is intended to be a collection of (hopefully helpful) ideas, but it will never take the place of an actual doctor-patient consultation.]

When you envision yourself having your procedure, you might imagine walking into a clinic or hospital and emerging a few hours later with fresh, glowing skin, a washboard tummy or more enhanced breasts. The reality is that, as with any surgery, you'll need time to recover both physically and mentally before you start enjoying noticeable results. We'll discuss the logistics of choosing a plastic surgeon and working with him or her in the planning and recovery phases, in Chapter 4.

Finally, in Chapter 5 we'll develop a "plan of approach" — going into detail to explore the many questions you will want to ask before you take the plunge. We break this down into easy, manageable steps, to help you get all the information you'll want to have, without being overwhelmed and frustrated. In the meantime, here are a few questions to help you decide whether you're ready for plastic surgery. Keep them in the back of your mind — as you read this book, as you share your thoughts with those you trust and as you do your own research to consider and compare different procedures and surgeons.

- Can any of my desired results be achieved solely through lifestyle changes like exercise, healthier eating, skin care, etc.?

- Do I want to see an improved version of my real self, or am I possibly trying to look like someone I'm not?

- Am I doing this because somebody else wants me to (more than I do)?

- Do I find myself becoming more anxious and worried thinking about a procedure, or more excited and happy?

You may not know all the answers right now, and that's okay. You're right at the beginning of your discovery! By reflecting on these questions as you go along, by the time you are ready to make a decision, you'll be much more likely to make the *right* decision for you.

Chapter 2: Is Plastic Surgery Right for You?

Many people, even those who are "basically happy" with how they look, are opting to undergo procedures to improve an aspect (or two) of their bodies. Often the cause is something over which they have no control, however the artistry and science of plastic surgery can help with. Let's first discuss the three main culprits that wage war on your natural, youthful beauty:

Genetics. You may have a natural tendency to accumulate fat in certain regions. Your skin may be especially prone to sun damage. Your breasts may not be proportionally matched to the rest of your body. Your nose might be unusually prominent, or your chin unusually weak. You can blame your parents for all these things, but there are procedures available now that can correct each one.

Gravity. The same force that makes a cup fall to the floor when you drop it is also hard at work on your body. Your tissues have been waging a valiant war against this force since you were born, but eventually, gravity wins. The cheeks that once sat high and proud on your face, begin to sag. The eyelids begin to droop. The breasts that once knew their proper place seem to be in a race toward the floor.

Age. Time itself is conspiring with gravity to diminish your good looks. As you age, your tissues become less resilient.

The skin is not as elastic, the muscles not as strong. They gradually lose their ability to retain your youthful form. At the same time, your skin is suffering the cumulative effects of sun exposure, which are permanent. And it doesn't replenish those skin cells as rapidly as it once did, so your skin may take on a gray, lifeless appearance.

Meanwhile, normal life events can make the problems worse. Pregnancy stretches the abdominal tissues, and they may not return to their pre-pregnancy state. The accompanying weight gain brings problems of its own. Stretch marks are common with pregnancy, and no matter what the skin cream manufacturers promise, they are permanent. If you've recently lost weight for any reason, it can be hard to celebrate your accomplishment when you still have excess loose skin. Other factors like illness, emotional stress and sun exposure can also accelerate the aging process. And if you're a smoker, here's one more reason to quit: smoking causes premature aging, in addition to inhibiting the healing process. Anyway, your surgeon will probably insist that you quit smoking before embarking on any major procedure. (And nicotine patches and gum won't help; it's the nicotine itself that's the culprit.)

So, armed with the right attitude and realistic expectations, let's explore the possibilities, benefits and potential drawbacks of plastic surgery. At the end of this chapter, you'll have a better idea of whether (and which) plastic surgery is right for you.

What plastic surgery is (and isn't)

First, plastic surgery is *not* the answer to certain problems. It's not a way to escape or change who you are as a person. Yes, your outside affects your inside, but this also holds true the other way around. For instance, if you're obsessed with a certain celebrity, and imagine that surgery will make you look just like her (or him), stop right here. The help you need won't be found in any physical transformation. Looks are important as far as how they can affect you emotionally, but should never be the basis for how you value yourself (or how anyone else values you). The truly beautiful women and men of the world understand this.

Some people feel dissatisfied with their bodies, when what they're not actually happy with is their overall identities. These issues are emotional, often with an underlying psychological component. And they're very normal; many of us have such insecurities, to some extent. The key is being able to recognize these issues and address them realistically, rather than chasing fantasies.

It's important to keep your expectations realistic. Plastic surgery will not transform an overweight person into a thin person. Some patients mistake plastic surgery for weight loss surgery. Having liposuction, for example, can contour your body and change your shape. It is not intended to be a weight reduction procedure. If you are truly obese, you likely need to lose weight *before* having plastic surgery.

If you're in your sixties, a well done procedure can make you look like you're in your forties... not your twenties. (And anyway, do you really want to look twenty-something forever? There are advantages to maturity and experience, after all!) Having unrealistic goals, or using plastic surgery as a "quick fix" for serious personal problems are what lead to some of the freakish cases we've all seen — people who've had so much work done that they barely look human. An ethical plastic surgeon will recognize such pathologies and direct patients to seek more appropriate remedies, such as lifestyle changes or counseling.

If you do it, do it for *you!*

As you weigh your options, here's another question to answer: are you trying to please someone other than yourself? Many people fear their partners will no longer find them attractive as they age; one patient spoke of having her breasts augmented "for" her boyfriend. Again, alarm bells should be going off. Even if your partner wants you to "have some work done," that's certainly not a good reason to do it. And even if you do it for them, it can backfire: the patient was pleased with her results, though her boyfriend felt that she should have gone even *bigger.* She realized (belatedly, but still rightly) that the decision wasn't up to him, and that pleasing herself was what gave her the sense of beauty and confidence she'd been seeking.

Doctor's Note
The least satisfied patients are those with unrealistic goals or body dysmorphic disorder — the patient who walks in and you know five minutes into it, that you can't ever make them happy. We develop very good antennae for that.

Sometimes people can get caught up in the details of who's paying for the surgery. If your partner is contributing financially in any way, that still does not give him or her the right to have a "say" over your body. You are not a car or a custom-built home; you are a person with autonomy over yourself. Anyone who attempts to pressure you emotionally or financially cannot be trusted as a reliable source of judgment.

Some people aren't sure whom they're trying to please. They've absorbed arbitrary standards of beauty from the culture, and think they have to look a certain way to be treated well or taken seriously. If that's you, all the more reason to step back and reconsider. The decision to have plastic surgery will require a clear head and rational cost-benefit analysis, using both your mind and your heart. Ultimately, you must decide based on your own needs and wishes. After all, it's your body; you're in control of it.

The best candidate for plastic surgery is a person who is happy, healthy — and realistic. She looks in the mirror with an objective eye, and identifies specific areas that could benefit from cosmetic enhancements. *She's not trying to become someone else*, but simply *the best possible version of herself.* With that in mind, she selects certain procedures to accomplish those goals, and sets her expectations accordingly.

She also seeks those enhancements that will look as natural as possible, and won't be glaringly obvious. One smart strategy is to have a little work done at a time, rather than trying to accomplish everything at once. You can view plastic surgery as part of an ongoing maintenance program, not a one-time cure-all. Doing it incrementally also allows you to assess the effectiveness of individual procedures as you go. The *extreme makeover* is an outdated concept, and for good reason. You can probably name several celebrities who *had work done* — and came out looking like totally different people. That's a tragic result that was all too common in years past. You can avoid it by taking small steps instead of giant leaps. One plastic surgeon tells his patients, "The only thing better than more is less."

What's your budget?

Finally, there's the financial aspect of plastic surgery. There are many non- and minimally invasive procedures that are quite affordable for most people, which can produce excellent results. A laser treatment to remove unwanted hair or spider veins may cost a few hundred dollars. But liposuction, breast augmentation, nose surgery, facelifts and tummy tucks are all serious surgical procedures; they are an investment in yourself and typically cost thousands of dollars. Remember, cosmetic procedures are considered elective, and so are not covered by health insurance. That should be a guide for you as well: your procedure may be important to you, but it's still a discretionary expense. If you're having trouble making the home mortgage payments, you probably need to hold off on plastic surgery.

That said, there are often payment plans available for cosmetic procedures (which most plastic surgeons offer). Before agreeing to such an arrangement, be realistic in assessing your ability to take on additional monthly payments for a surgical procedure. Consider how long you'll be making the payments and what the interest rates will be. One of the most popular financing companies for elective cosmetic procedures is Care Credit, which can be found at www.CareCredit.com.

Sometimes a cosmetic procedure can be combined with another one that *is* medically necessary, and thus be partially paid for by insurance. A large part of the expense of surgery is in securing the facility, the anesthesiologist, etc. If those expenses are covered for one procedure, you may be able to include another at the same time and save money. For example, if you have breathing problems (deviated septum) but would also like to improve the outer appearance of your nose, you could combine these into one operation — a septo/rhinoplasty. This way you are treating the functional airway issue and the cosmetic concern at the same time. The septoplasty portion may be covered by your health insurance and the rhinoplasty would be paid for out of pocket. Since insurance plans vary greatly in coverage, discuss this in more detail with your surgeon and your health insurance carrier in advance.

It's important to get the most accurate cost estimate possible. A surgeon may quote his or her surgeon's fee, but a detailed estimate may include the cost of the facility and materials, the anesthesiologist's fee, surgical garments (if needed), lab work, medications and follow-up visits. If revision surgery is needed, who will pay for that? You should discuss all these things candidly with your physician, and make sure you have a clear idea of *all* the costs before you proceed. You may want to look for online reviews and testimonials from other people who've had the same (or a similar) procedure performed either by your surgeon or by someone else in a geographic area similar to yours (since costs can vary by location).

Chapter 3: Mirror, Mirror...
Selecting a Procedure (or Two)

Look in the mirror. Really *look*. Don't critique and don't judge; you're simply observing. What do you see?

First, identify the features of your face and/or body you like best. What's good about them? How do they reflect who you really are?

Now, identify the areas that you're least happy with. What do you want to change or restore? Itemize these and rank them in order of importance.

Chances are, there are procedures that can address most of them. If you're having trouble being objective at this point, the judgment of an experienced plastic surgeon can be invaluable. Your surgeon deals with these issues every day, and has a better vantage point to make reality-based observations. He or she can tell you what can and cannot be realistically done, take detailed measurements/photos and answer all your questions (as well as those you didn't know you had).

There is, of course, much more to choosing the right surgeon than a simple Google search, but the reason you probably picked up this book in the first place was to find out more about the process and possibilities of each type of procedure. So let's get started!

The following information is not an exhaustive description of what's available, or of the risks involved. For more detailed information, you should research the areas you're interested in, and of course, consult with a plastic surgeon. But this will give you an overview of some of the most popular cosmetic procedures. "Invasive" procedures are surgeries that typically require a general anesthetic or IV sedation. For these procedures you are either completely asleep or partially asleep. There are also "non-invasive" and "minimally invasive" procedures, such as chemical peels and Botox; these are generally performed while you're awake. Non-invasive procedures, by definition, are non-surgical and involve no incisions whatsoever. Minimally invasive procedures involve only tiny incisions or injections.

Invasive procedures (surgery)

Let's start with the part of your body that you — and everyone else — looks at the most.

Face and Neck

Facelift (rhytidectomy): Over time, the skin of your neck and lower face begins to sag. You may lose skin elasticity and muscle tone in your face and neck, developing jowls and deep creases. The soft tissue of the face also begins to atrophy with aging, causing a flattened, deflated look. Fat transfer to the face is often performed at the same time as a facelift to restore lost volume. A facelift will remove this excess skin and tighten other tissues, restoring a more youthful look. It can improve the nasolabial folds — the creases that extend from your nose down each side of your mouth. It can also alleviate jowls and a sagging platysma (that muscle in your neck that sometimes hangs loose after a certain age). Neck fat may also be removed. The incision for a facelift starts above your ear, going down the front of the ear around the earlobe, up the back of the ear and into the hairline behind the ear. There will be another small incision beneath your chin. You can conceal the incisions with makeup two weeks after the procedure, and the scars will begin to fade in three to six months' time.

Most patients report mild discomfort after a facelift — usually described as a "tight" feeling in the face, as well as swelling and bruising that can last up to two weeks.

Afterward, you'll not only enjoy a smoother, more youthful appearance, but you'll probably find you feel more energetic, more confident and happier with yourself overall, as people notice and wonder, "Wow! Something seems different about her... though I can't quite tell what." A good facelift is not obvious and can last up to ten years or more with proper self-care (healthy diet and exercise, regular skincare, etc.) You may decide (as millions of others have) that it's well worth the inconvenience.

There are several variations and terminology used to describe facelifts: deep plane facelifts (subperiosteal), midface lifts, SMAS lift, mini-facelift — just to name a few. As you can see, all facelifts are not the same, so be sure your surgeon clearly outlines which procedure is best for you based upon your specific anatomy.

Neck lift (platysmaplasty). This involves tightening of the neck muscle (platysma) and removal of neck fat, but no removal of excess skin. The incision is located just underneath the chin and heals quite well. This procedure can create a more defined jawline in the right patient. A neck lift is typically combined with a facelift procedure but can be performed on its own in certain patients.

Brow lift. We use our forehead muscles to express a variety of emotions: surprise, joy, amusement, sympathy, anger and worry, to name a few. The wrinkles we develop there through repeated use can settle into a permanently sad, tired or angry expression. The brow itself will also tend to hang down over time. A forehead lift, also known as a brow lift, can improve the brow position and alleviate wrinkles. In the hands of a skilled surgeon, the effect can be dramatic. In some cases, it can alter the appearance in unwanted ways; there may also be permanent hair loss at the scar line. Numbness can occur, which is usually temporary, but in rare cases is permanent.

Eyelid lift (*blepharoplasty*). This popular procedure involves removing the excess skin and fat in the upper and/or lower eyelids. Rejuvenation of the eyelids can have a profound impact on a person's face and needs to be performed carefully. You want to end up looking like a better version of yourself.

The risks include blindness (one in 10,000 cases), blurred or double vision (less than one percent, usually temporary), corneal abrasion (treatable), swelling of the whites of the eyes and eyelid linings, and various undesirable aesthetic effects.

Nose surgery (rhinoplasty). One of the most common cosmetic procedures performed in men and women. It alters primarily the bone and cartilage of the nose — the centerpiece of the face. Each rhinoplasty is customized to the anatomy and desires of each patient. That makes it important for you to know precisely what look you're looking for, and to communicate it clearly to your surgeon. Most nose surgery involves reducing the size of the nose, but a nose can also be enlarged, using implants of synthetic material or bone harvested from the patient's hip, ear or rib. There will be a small incision under the nose ("open" rhinoplasty) or inside the nose ("closed" rhinoplasty).

This can be performed on an outpatient basis with sedation or general anesthesia. It takes between one and three hours, and will be accompanied by swelling for two to four weeks. The tip of the nose may be numb for several weeks, and you may develop black eyes for the first week. Because the nose is so close to the brain, there are rare but serious potential risks, including leakage of cerebrospinal fluid, accumulation of air around the brain and meningitis. The revision surgery rate for rhinoplasty ranges from five to fifteen percent, depending on the surgeon. The benefits of a well done rhinoplasty can make you look and feel more symmetric, confident and happy.

In certain cases, rhinoplasty may be medically necessary (and thus covered by insurance) if a patient's nasal septum (the tissue separating left and right nasal passages) is crooked (deviated), making it hard to breathe.

Chin augmentation (genioplasty). If your chin is weak or underprojected, this procedure can give you a stronger profile. It involves cutting the chin bone, moving it forward and securing it with screws or wires. There is some risk of nerve damage and numbness.

Chin implants are another option used to augment a small chin. Implants are a less drastic procedure and don't require as much recovery time as genioplasty. The implant is typically made of a synthetic material like silicone. Incisions are made under the chin or inside the mouth. Complications are few but include numbness of the chin, infection of the implant or movement of the implant over time.

Cheek augmentation. This can be done on its own or combined with a facelift or chin surgery. Implants of bone or synthetic material are placed in the cheeks to produce a fuller, more rounded appearance. If you're having a facelift at the same time, the surgeon may implant your own tissue (fat) taken from other areas. Incisions are made in the mouth between cheeks and gums, at the lower eyelids or in front of the ears. As with all such implants, there is a risk of extrusion, infection and numbness of skin.

Otoplasty (ear pinning). Both men and women can be self-conscious about the size of their ears. About five percent of the population has large or noticeable ears (also known as prominent ears). An ear pinning procedure (otoplasty) can bring the ears closer to the head by removing and reshaping the ear cartilage. This is typically done at any age after the age of six or seven years old up into adulthood. The procedure involves an incision made behind the ear, where the ear meets the scalp. The scar heals very well as it blends into the natural crease behind the ear. The surgery takes about an hour or two and is performed under sedation or general anesthesia. The results are seen immediately and patients report a very high satisfaction rate.

Ask Dr. Bruno*

Question: At what age is a facelift appropriate?

Dr. Bruno: As patients age, the facial skin and soft tissue begins to sag and atrophy (shrink). Some people may have loose skin of their neck and lower face with jowls, and also a sunken appearance in the cheek/lower eyelid area. Most patients only need a small amount of skin removal — what they really need is for the soft tissue under their skin to be elevated and repositioned.

At the same time, many patients also need a fat transfer to this area to restore some of the lost volume. Usually the best time to have a facelift is *before you really need* a facelift. This could be in the early forties, or sometime in the fifties. The age is not as important as the quality of their skin and soft tissue position. As always, I urge patients to please consult with a board-certified plastic surgeon prior to scheduling this or any procedure.

Question: I cannot afford to miss very much work after blepharoplasty. What is the standard eyelid surgery recovery time?

Dr. Bruno: Most patients will require about one week off of work from either upper or lower (or both) eyelid surgery. This is due to the visible bruising that may persist for about seven days or so. The pain is not significant, with most patients taking oral pain medications for only two or three days. Usually the stitches are removed on the sixth or seventh day. In women, if there is some residual bruising, this can usually be concealed with some cover-up makeup.

As long as your plastic surgeon is very careful with controlling the blood loss during the surgery, the bruising is usually very well tolerated in most patients. Frequent ice packs to the eye area for the first day or two also helps minimize the bruising and swelling.

Question: Will I have visible scars from a nose job? If I have a problem with keloids, am I still a candidate?

Dr. Bruno: There are two types of rhinoplasties: open and closed. In an open approach, there is a small incision made on the columella, which is the part of the nose between the nostrils. This heals very well and is virtually undetectable in most cases. A closed rhinoplasty involves no external incisions, with all the incisions located inside the nostrils. The open approach allows for better exposure, especially if more intricate work is to be done on the nasal tip or a patient requires a revision.

The scar usually heals remarkably well on the nose after a rhinoplasty. Keloids (thick, raised scars) do not typically form in this area and are not usually a concern after a rhinoplasty. If you are prone to keloids in other areas of your body (chest, shoulder, ear), let your plastic surgeon know prior to surgery.

In all cases, ask your board-certified surgeon to show you photos of this incision and to discuss the options available to you for rhinoplasty techniques.

*Always consult your doctor before having any procedures or treatments

Breasts

Ok, now for the *second* thing people notice… no, just kidding. But there is a very good reason that breast augmentation remains the second most popular type of plastic surgery (after liposuction). After all, while most of us don't seek facial plastic surgery until later in life, women of all ages can enjoy the benefits of a firmer, fuller bust. Whether you're looking to increase the size of your breasts and/or give them a bit more lift, or even if you want them reduced, there are several options.

Breast augmentation. The first question is usually: how much volume/size is appropriate? You must decide for yourself what is healthy and natural-looking, but ideally, the final results should look proportional for your body type. A surgeon may help you decide by having you try on sizers, which you can wear with a sports bra, to get an idea what various sizes look and feel like. Some doctors may use computerized imaging to simulate what you may look like. Remember that breast implants are measured by volume in cubic centimeters (cc), and not by cup size (which isn't actually a standardized measurement). Your surgeon will estimate how many cc's are required to reach a certain bra cup size.

Augmentation can be performed in several different ways:

Silicone implants. These have been around the longest. Ever since being re-approved by the FDA in 2006, they are better than ever before — and safe. Modern silicone implants consist of a strong but flexible solid silicone shell. The silicone filler is about the consistency of a gummy bear candy. It's lighter than saline, and looks and feels more natural.

Silicone implants are more durable than saline and have a significantly lower rupture rate compared to saline implants. The best way to detect a ruptured silicone breast implant is by way of an MRI, which is recommended three years after surgery, then every two years thereafter. (Mammograms and ultrasounds are not very sensitive at detecting silicone implant ruptures).

Saline implants. First, the bad news... saline implants are heavier than silicone, and are thus more prone to sagging. They tend to feel stiffer, and can assume an unnaturally

Before

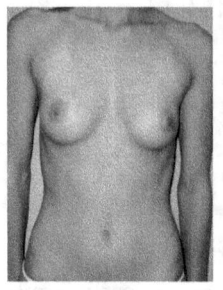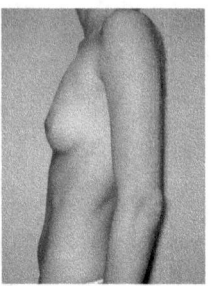

After

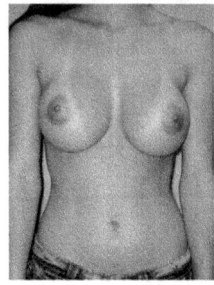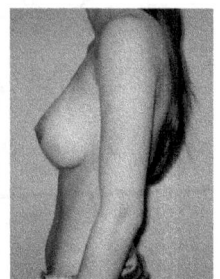

25-year-old woman before (top)
and after (bottom) 375-cc
silicone breast augmentation

round appearance. Occasionally, the edges of the implant can be seen through the skin or felt, which is referred to as rippling or wrinkling. This rippling phenomenon is more commonly seen in thin patients with very little breast tissue who undergo saline breast augmentation. Saline implants are also filled after they're inserted, so slightly smaller incisions are required. They generally deflate at a rate of approximately one percent each year. Deflations occur more commonly with saline implants but are easier to detect than silicone implant ruptures. In the event of a

Before

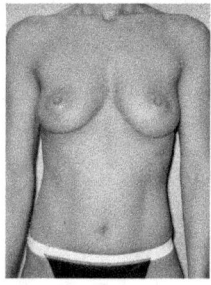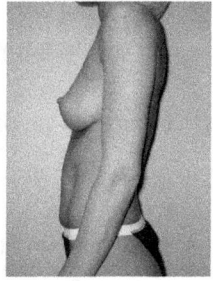

After

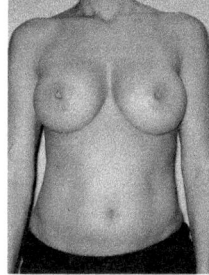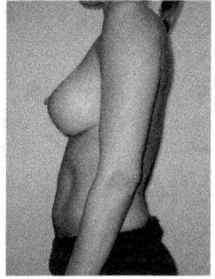

38-year-old woman before (left)
and after (right) 375-cc
silicone breast augmentation

ruptured or deflated saline breast implant, your body will simply absorb the saline, which is merely salt water.

So which is right for you — saline or silicone? Silicone implants are more popular, even though they are slightly more expensive. They're more durable and natural looking (and feeling!) The FDA recommends that patients be twenty-two years of age to be eligible for silicone breast implants — for cosmetic reasons. Saline implants are less expensive, though they feel less "natural" to the touch. There's also a greater chance of saline implants deflating over time. Contrary to what you may have heard, the myth of needing to replace breast implants every ten years is just that — a myth.

Let's briefly review some of the more common complications and side effects of breast augmentation.

Capsular contracture is the term for hard scar tissue that can form around breast implants. This occurs in about ten to fifteen percent of all patients who undergo breast augmentation. The implants can feel hard to the touch, and in severe cases can look asymmetric or distorted. This happens more often with implants inserted through the areola and implants placed in front of (above) the pectoral muscle. In addition to massaging your implants after surgery, there are some medications that can alleviate this problem. If the scar tissue becomes painful, patients may require surgery to remove the scar tissue and replace the implants.

Nipple sensation changes can occur after breast augmentation. It's possible you might lose sensation or experience decreased sensation in your nipples. This happens in about ten percent of cases. The majority of patients regain their normal nipple sensation within a few weeks to months after surgery.

Breastfeeding is possible in the majority of patients after breast augmentation. There are certain approaches that may increase the likelihood of being able to breastfeed, such as, the inframammary incision (under the breast). There are no known risks to infants of breastfeeding from women with saline or silicone breast implants.

Mammograms are still recommended in women with breast implants. There are special mammographic techniques available for women with implants to obtain the best image possible. Still, breast implants may prevent about ten percent of the breast tissue from being visualized on a mammogram. Therefore, a potential mass or cancer could be obscured by a breast implant. An MRI study could give a more detailed image, if necessary in certain cases.

Incisions may be placed under the breast (inframammary), around the nipple (periareolar), under the armpit (axilla) or in the belly button (umbilical). The scars are typically hidden and take about six to twelve months to heal completely. The procedure takes one hour, and is typically performed on an outpatient basis in a surgery center or physician's office. Mild to severe discomfort may last from three to seven days, and can be alleviated by prescription pain medications. Most patients take about three to four days off from work to recover. Strenuous activity is avoided for about four to six weeks after surgery. The implants will take about two months to "settle" — they look high on the chest wall at first but lower and softer with time. A surgical bra or sports bra is worn for the first month after surgery.

Either type of implant may be placed either above the pectoral muscle (subglandular) or under the muscle (subpectoral/submuscular). Subglandular involves less discomfort and faster recovery, but there's also a greater risk of capsular contracture. The implants may be more likely to shift downward, and to interfere with mammograms. Placement under the muscle (submuscular) will involve more pain and swelling, and a longer recovery. However, submuscular implants tend to look more natural, have lower capsular contracture rates, higher breastfeeding rates and better mammogram images.

Before

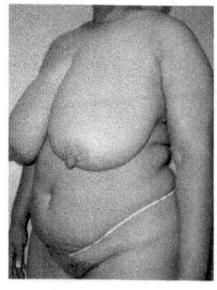 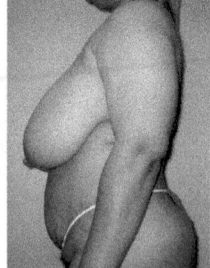

After

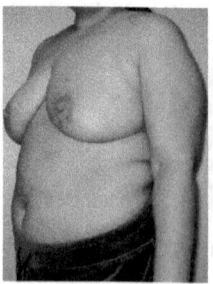 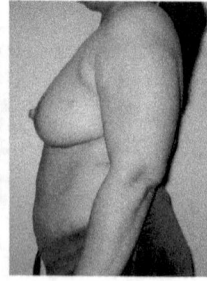

40-year-old woman before (top)
and after (bottom)
breast reduction

Before

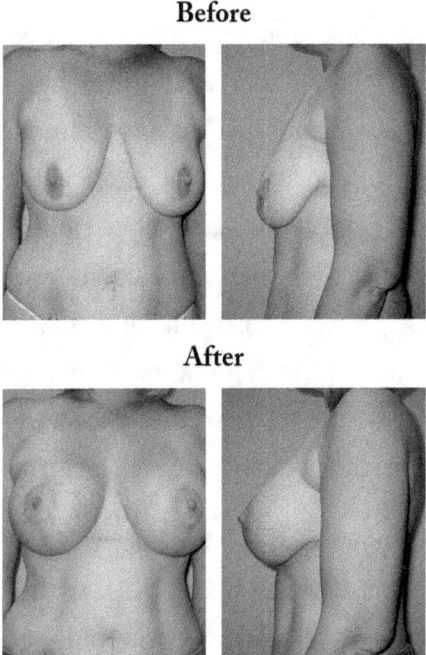

After

38-year-old woman before (top)
and after (bottom) breast
lift with 371-cc augmentation

Fat transfer to the breast (fat graft). Some women want to increase their breast size without the use of saline or silicone implants. This can be accomplished in certain cases through the use of a fat transfer procedure. Fat is liposuctioned from various areas of your body (for example, the abdomen or thighs), purified and injected into the breasts to create a firmer, fuller look and feel. A single cup size is generally the maximum effect you'll be able to achieve with this procedure. The procedure can take anywhere from three to four hours and is done under general anesthesia.

Be aware, however, that fat grafts come with their own risks: the fat can dissolve and be reabsorbed over time (about fifty percent of the fat will shrink/atrophy in the first few months), or become lumpy, as your immune system tries to "wall off" the fatty material (called a granulomatous reaction). This granuloma leads to calcium formation, and calcium formation is what radiologists are screening for when looking for breast cancer. Therefore, fat grafting to the breasts can make interpretation of mammograms more difficult. Some of the fat that does not survive can develop into oil cysts that may require drainage or excision.

Breast lift (mastopexy). If you are happy with the size of your breasts but want a better shape, a breast lift may be right for you. Breast skin and breast tissue can sag due to gravity, aging and pregnancy. A breast lift is a great way to remove excess skin, elevate the nipple position and decrease the size of the areolas (if needed). A properly done breast lift can create a perkier breast and improved shape. Some patients may benefit from a small breast implant at the time of their breast lift for added volume and fullness. There are a variety of breast lift techniques available and your plastic surgeon can recommend the best one for you based on your anatomy. This is an outpatient procedure involving sedation or general anesthesia. It takes between one and three hours, and you can be back to work in three to four days. As with other surgeries, you can expect mild to moderate discomfort for a week or two; swelling and bruising may persist for three to ten days.

Breast reduction (reduction mammoplasty). You may need reduction mammoplasty if your breasts are heavy enough to cause neck and/or back pain. When the breasts are heavy enough to cause these issues, health insurance may cover breast reduction surgery. Not only will a breast reduction make your breasts smaller and lighter, it will also allow for a "lift" as well, improving their shape. The recovery from a breast reduction is similar to that of a breast lift — plan to take about three or four days off from work.

Ask Dr. Bruno*

Question: I'm considering breast augmentation. How big is too big?

Dr. Bruno: This is a difficult question to answer, but there are a few studies to suggest that implants over 400cc may be associated with more complications. This does not mean you should not have an implant over that size, because there are many variables that need to be considered (skin quality, breast tissue, body habitus). You need to examine several implants and review the sizes in detail with your board-certified plastic surgeon prior to insertion. The implant should be suited to your anatomy and body proportion. Larger breast implants are heavier and therefore may sag more over time.

Question: What is the recovery period like for breast augmentation?

Dr. Bruno: The vast majority of patients can recover from breast augmentation within three days, provided their work doesn't involve heavy lifting. Most patients who do office work for example, and have surgery on a Friday, can return to work by Monday, as they are usually off the narcotic pain medication within seventy-two hours. However, some patients may need a few additional days of pain medication before they feel comfortable returning to work.

Regardless of your occupation, you should avoid heavy lifting or strenuous activity with your arms for about four to six weeks if your implants are placed under the pectoral muscle.

Question: What can I expect during a breast lift recovery?

Dr. Bruno: The recovery from a breast lift (mastopexy) is not as involved as the recovery from breast augmentation. Since most breast lifts require removal of skin and tissue *only* (the muscle is left intact) patients can return to work in two to three days.

Prescription oral pain medication is required for only two to three days, after which time patients can return to work and drive while taking just Tylenol. A surgical bra or sports bra is usually worn for about four weeks after the procedure.

Question: How long will my breast lift last?

Dr. Bruno: It is difficult to answer this question because there are so many variables involved with breast lifts (skin quality, breast tissue, type of procedure, age of patient, etc.)

In general, a mastopexy can be expected to last ten to twenty years, provided you maintain your body weight and wear bras more often than not. A pregnancy after a breast lift could compromise your result and leave you in a position where you need a second procedure to correct your nipple position and improve your breast shape.

Question: Can I get implants at the same time as a breast lift?

Dr. Bruno: It depends. If your breasts are fairly large or fairly ptotic (sagging), then it makes sense to do the procedures in two separate stages. Generally the breast lift is done first, and then a few months later the implants can be inserted. This is safer from a blood supply standpoint, and tends to give a more predictable result cosmetically. It really depends a lot on your specific anatomy. If your breasts are smaller or atrophied from pregnancy, then a combined, one-stage procedure is possible. I would consult with a few board-certified plastic surgeons who are experienced in this particular area of breast surgery.

Question: When can I start working out my chest again after male breast reduction surgery?

Dr. Bruno: A male breast reduction usually involves liposuction of the chest and direct removal of breast tissue, and occasionally some skin. Patients must wear a compressive garment or vest after the surgery for about four weeks to help with contour and swelling. I advise patients to avoid heavy lifting or strenuous upper body exercise for about four to six weeks after surgery. This will help reduce any shearing forces or stress of the chest soft tissue against the pectoral muscle.

You may resume aerobic exercise (running, cycling, etc.) in about one week.

*Always consult your doctor before having any procedures or treatments.

Body

And now for the rest of you!

Liposuction. The number one procedure that men and women seek is liposuction, which has been around since the 1970s. Liposuction has been extensively studied at the basic science level as well as in numerous clinical trials by plastic surgeons and dermatologists. Both traditional and minimally invasive liposuction techniques can permanently remove existing fat cells, creating better shapes and body contours.

The difference between "traditional" and "minimally invasive" liposuction depends on the size of the liposuction cannulas (metal tubes) and the type of suctioning used. Medical advancements and the use of assistive energy (vibration, laser, ultrasound, etc.) have allowed the use of smaller cannulas, but many people still choose to have a traditional procedure. If you're considering liposuction, it is extremely important that you discuss the options in detail with your doctor, but we can go over the general aspects of both here.

It is important to understand that liposuction is not a substitute for diet and exercise, and those who view it as a shortcut to a desired weight are likely to be disappointed. If you've been gaining weight, you'll probably keep doing so after liposuction. And if you're losing weight, you should wait till your weight is stable before considering it. The ideal candidate for liposuction is someone who has reached an acceptable weight, but still has particular areas where fat accumulation persists. Younger patients with good skin tone will see the best results. For women, the areas most commonly treated with liposuction are the abdomen, flanks (love handles), back, hips, thighs, knees, arms and neck. The rate of revision surgery is between five and fifteen percent.

It is also important to know that liposuction, whether traditional or minimally invasive, is a serious procedure that carries potential risks. Lidocaine toxicity may result from excessive infiltration of the tissues with the tumescent solution (a watery solution used to extract the fat). Blood clots or fat emboli can develop and travel to the lungs causing a pulmonary embolus. There may be excessive bruising in some cases. The most common side effect or complication of liposuction is that of contour irregularities. This basically means the skin can have an uneven appearance with some visible indentations. This phenomenon occurs in about ten percent of liposuction cases.

Also, liposuction does *not* eliminate cellulite. Most liposuction procedures deal with the deep fat layers, while cellulite occurs in the superficial layers.

After anesthesia is administered, the surgeon will usually make a few small incisions and then inject fluid, which aids in the removal of the fat cells. The surgeon will then insert the metal cannula under the skin and move it around the affected area, literally sucking out the fatty tissue. The higher the volume of fat removed, the greater the risk, the more blood loss and the more need for anesthetic.

The procedure may take anywhere from thirty minutes to a few hours, depending on the size of the patient and number of areas treated. It can be performed in a hospital or office, with local or general anesthesia. It can be an outpatient procedure, but high-volume liposuction (more than five liters of fat) may require an overnight stay. Expect mild-to-severe discomfort for three to seven days, treatable with prescription pain medication. Depending on your procedure, bruising will persist for seven to ten days, and swelling should resolve after four to six weeks. You may feel numbness and tingling for a few weeks. And final visible results might not be seen for about three months. You'll probably need to wear a liposuction garment for several weeks, to support and apply pressure to the suctioned areas, and to promote skin retraction. Your surgeon will typically provide you with a garment at the time of surgery. You may want to get two, so you'll have one to wear while the other is in the wash.

Ask Dr. Bruno*

Question: Who should perform liposuction? Can any doctor do it, or would I need to see a specialist of some kind?

Dr. Bruno: Liposuction should be performed by a board-certified plastic surgeon, preferably a member of the American Society of Plastic Surgeons (ASPS) or the American Society for Aesthetic Plastic Surgery (ASAPS). These surgeons typically have the most training and experience necessary to perform the procedure with best results and fewest complications. Board-certified dermatologists may also perform this procedure.

Although non-plastic surgeons can legally perform liposuction, that may not be their specialty, and they may have only taken minimal training (like a weekend course) to learn it. Be careful when choosing a physician to perform your liposuction procedure.

Question: What are the potential liposuction side effects?

Dr. Bruno: The most common side effect after liposuction is an irregular contour to the skin. There can be uneven areas with some minor depressions or bumps if the suctioning is performed too close to the surface of the skin or if the patient's skin has poor elasticity or stretch marks. The incidence of having a small area of irregular contour is about ten percent, but this varies depending upon skin tone and surgeon technique. Sometimes this can be corrected by performing a fat transfer to "fill in" a small depressed area. However, if an area has significant irregularity, it may not be correctable. Other less common side effects include temporary numbness, asymmetry, poor scarring or prolonged bruising.

Question: How many areas can you treat in one liposuction session?

Dr. Bruno: For outpatient liposuction, five liters (just under 170 fluid ounces) of fat is considered the maximum amount that can be safely removed in one session. During that session, several different areas can be addressed, from one area up to four or five. However, if a patient is requesting or needs many areas (more than five), then serious consideration should be given to perhaps losing more weight prior to the liposuction surgery. Some patients are under the false impression that liposuction is a means for them to lose weight; this is not true. The goal of liposuction is to improve contour, not to lower weight.

As always, please consult with a board-certified plastic surgeon prior to considering liposuction or any other plastic surgery.

*Always consult your doctor before having any procedures or treatments.

Body Contouring Surgeries

As helpful as liposuction is, it only addresses the issue of fat accumulation. As we've seen, another source of trouble for many people is loose saggy skin, which gets worse with age and is especially troublesome after dramatic weight fluctuations. Many patients who have had weight loss surgery (Lap Band, gastric sleeve, gastric bypass) end up with significant areas of loose skin which needs to be addressed.

Arm lift (brachioplasty). As with other types of "lift" procedures, this one is best for removing loose skin (rather than fat) from the back of the arm area. If fat deposits are also a problem, liposuction may also be performed as part of the procedure. The incision is placed along the inside of the arm, from elbow to armpit, and is a great way to remove that excess "bat wing" skin commonly seen in certain patients.

Buttock Augmentation: Fat vs Implants

Fat transfer to the buttock (Brazilian butt lift). This procedure involves removing fat from one or more areas of the body and redistributing it to the buttock/hip area. Fat is liposuctioned from various locations of your body (usually the abdomen,

thighs or love handles), purified and then injected into the buttocks/hips. Depending on how thin you are, you may even want to *gain* a little weight for this procedure. (Win-win!) A properly done buttock augmentation with fat can create a very attractive waist-to-hip ratio while simultaneously increasing the size of your buttock. This is a great way to removed fat from unwanted areas (for example, the abdomen) and transfer it to more desirable areas (for example, the buttock). The majority of the injected fat will become permanent;

however, about one-third of the fat will shrink and atrophy in the first few months after surgery.

Before

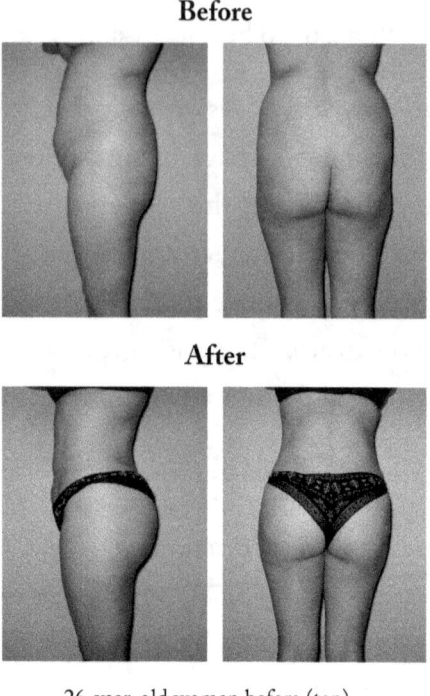

After

26-year-old woman before (top)
and after (bottom)
600-cc Brazilian butt lift

Although a fat transfer to the buttock is quite safe, there are some risks you should be aware of as a patient. Some known complications of a Brazilian buttock lift include: fatty necrosis (hard scar tissue from atrophied fat), fat emboli (fat that can travel to the lungs), injury to the sciatic nerve, deep vein thrombosis (DVT or blood clot), seromas (fluid collections), and infection. Be sure to discuss these with your doctor in advance.

Although you may feel ready to get back to work and resume normal activity a few days after surgery, you will need to spend about one to two weeks resting. It is imperative that you do not put any weight on your buttocks during this time, because the new fat cells can be easily damaged. You can use a modified pillow placed under the backs of your thighs for assistance with sitting for the first three to four weeks. For the first four weeks, patients will wear a compression garment to limit swelling. After four weeks, most of the obvious swelling will be gone and you will be able to remove the garment.

The longer you avoid directly sitting on your buttocks, the better result you will have. Keep your weight stable and avoid strenuous exercise for eight weeks after surgery. Fat burning exercises can effectively kill the fat cells injected into your butt. Skipping exercise for a few months will ensure that an essential blood supply is established to the new fat cells, improving their survival. Results are usually final within four to six months.

Buttock Implants. An alternative to using your body's own fat is to use a silicone implant to increase the size of your buttocks. This option is typically reserved for those patients who simply do not have enough fat on their body to have a fat transfer procedure. Gluteal implants, however, tend to look and feel less natural compared to a fat transfer. These implants also have higher complications and surgical revision rates.

Thigh lift. If you have loose, excess skin of your inner thigh area, then a thigh lift procedure may be a good option. This surgery is usually indicated in patients who have experienced significant weight loss. The incision can be placed near the crease of the groin, but in some cases may also require an extension along the inside of the thigh to the knee. Although the scar may be visible, the improved contour and thigh shape is worth it to most patients.

Tummy tuck (abdominoplasty). By far the most commonly performed of the body contouring surgeries. A tummy tuck is usually performed in patients that have had multiple pregnancies or who have experienced significant weight fluctuations throughout life. This procedure can create a very dramatic impact on a woman's body by addressing excess skin/fat, stretch marks and a weakened abdominal wall (bulge). By tightening the abdominal muscles that become stretched with pregnancy, the "abs" are repositioned back to their correct anatomic location — creating a flat abdomen. The excess skin and stretch marks from belly button to pubic area also removed completely. In most cases, some liposuction of the flanks (love handles) is done at the same time, to further accentuate the waistline.

A tummy tuck usually takes about two to three hours to perform, and in most cases is done under general anesthesia. There will typically be two drains left under the skin to help remove excess fluid and prevent a seroma (fluid collection). These drains are removed about one week after surgery.

You'll also wear an abdominal binder or garment for four to six weeks. You should avoid a tummy tuck if you are obese or a smoker, or are anticipating future pregnancies. A good plastic surgeon will be able to examine you and determine if you are a good candidate for this procedure.

Before

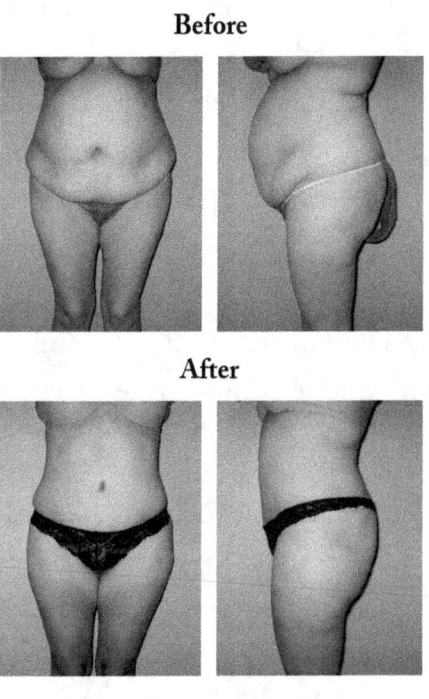

After

40-year-old woman before (top)
and after (bottom)
tummy tuck with liposuction of the flanks

A *mini* tummy tuck removes only some of the excess skin of the lower abdomen, and does not allow for complete tightening of the abdominal wall. Mini tummy tucks are usually done in very thin patients who have only a small amount of loose skin of their lower abdominal area.

Tummy tucks (and mini-tummy tucks) have risks and complications as any surgery. The most important risk to be aware of, however, is that of a deep vein thrombosis (DVT) that can progress to a pulmonary embolus (PE). Basically, this means a blood clot can form in your legs during or after the surgery, and migrate to your lungs and become life-threatening. Although this risk is quite low (one to three percent), it's important to take measures to prevent it. Compression stockings, compression devices during surgery, early walking after surgery, avoidance of smoking and birth control pills — are a few worth mentioning. Other common side effects of a tummy tuck include numbness of the lower/mid abdomen (which can be permanent), a thick scar (keloid) or an irregular shape to the end of the scar ("dog ears").

There are also some variations on the tummy tuck that you may come across in your research. A "body lift", for example, usually involves a tummy tuck with an extension around the back of the body — also known as a "circumferential body lift". This surgery is generally done in patients who have had massive weight loss. Another type of tummy tuck commonly seen is a called a "Fleur-de-lis tummy tuck", which adds a vertical incision to the traditional tummy tuck incision. This allows for removal of excess skin of the mid/upper abdomen in certain patients.

Ask Dr. Bruno*

Question: If I get an arm lift, how long would the results of the surgery last? Would there be anything that could happen that would make the saggy skin on my arms come back after the arm lift?

Dr. Bruno: If you maintain your weight after an arm lift (brachioplasty), the results will be long-lasting. It's difficult to say the results will be "permanent" because skin is constantly undergoing changes due to gravity and the aging process. However, if performed properly in a good candidate, the results should last for many years. The most important factor is to be at a stable body weight, before and after the procedure, so your skin laxity does not change significantly.

Most patients are quite pleased with this procedure. However, you must be willing to accept the scars, which can take up to a year or longer to fade.

Question: I know it depends greatly on the individual, but which arm lift scar is favored by most women?

Dr. Bruno: The location of the scar for an arm lift (brachioplasty) varies depending on a patient's anatomy and skin laxity. Generally, the scar is located on the medial or inner aspect of the arm, extending from the elbow to the armpit. Sometimes this scar can be located slightly more posteriorly, or toward the back of the arm. The goal is to provide a good contour while at the same time concealing the scar when the arm is down by the patient's side. Regardless of where the scar is located, patients must realize that the scar can potentially be permanently dark in color and may be slightly thick. This is a trade-off, meaning you will have a better contour, but may have a noticeable scar.

Question: Which will give sufficient lift, volume and shape to the bottom, a Brazilian buttock augmentation or a butt injection?

Dr. Bruno: A Brazilian buttock lift and a fat transfer to the buttock are essentially the same thing. This involves liposuction of the lower back, sides (flanks) and sometimes abdomen to harvest and remove unwanted fat. Then, the fat is prepared and strained, and only the pure fat (without blood or fluid) is injected deep into the gluteal area to provide a fuller look to the buttocks.

This creates a larger appearing buttock, with the liposuction of the lower back and sides, and gives a very aesthetically appealing gluteal/lower back/waist line appearance.

The ideal patient for this procedure is someone who is in good health/shape but has a little extra fat; that fat is necessary in order to transfer it to the gluteal area.

Question: What is the best scar placement with a thigh lift?

Dr. Bruno: There are two types of scars used for a thigh lift. A horizontal scar placed in the groin crease is best for patients who have significant vertical laxity (loose skin which can easily be pulled upward). A vertical incision along the inner aspect of the thigh from groin to knee is best used if you have significant horizontal skin laxity or looseness. The specific incision needs to be tailored to your specific anatomy.

I would add that the scars can migrate or widen from their original position; something patients should be made aware of before their surgery.

I recommend consulting with a board-certified plastic surgeon that is experienced in this type of body contouring procedure.

Question: Will losing weight after a tummy tuck lead to flabby skin?

Dr. Bruno: If you lose a lot of weight after a tummy tuck, you may be left with some loose skin and a contour that is not as nice as the day of surgery. You would need to lose the weight very gradually in order to minimize the amount of loose skin. You should discuss this in greater detail with your plastic surgeon before having your procedure done.

Question: I am having a body lift in five days and just stopped smoking today. Will five days smoke-free prior to surgery aid in my recovery, as long as I continue not to smoke afterward?

Dr. Bruno: You should stop smoking at least two to three weeks before and after *any* plastic surgery procedure, including body contouring surgery. Smoking can increase your wound healing complications and infection rates.

Also, smoking can increase your chances of developing a blood clot in your lower extremities (a deep vein thrombosis, or DVT). Please obtain medical clearance from your primary care physician prior to scheduling your procedure. You should also be honest with your plastic surgeon about how long you have been smoke-free prior to having a body lift or body contouring procedure.

*Always consult your doctor before having any procedures or treatments.

Mommy Makeover

Does being a mother involve doing whatever is necessary for the welfare of your children? Of course it does. Without question. Does being a mother mean your social life ends and you're no longer concerned with yourself and your appearance? Absolutely not.

Most women want to get their pre-pregnancy body back and to feel as beautiful as possible. A post-pregnancy exercise plan and healthy diet are important, of course, but sometimes more assistance is needed. You've given life to a brand new human being. You deserve a bit of a break! Combining several procedures into one surgery — commonly referred to as a "mommy makeover" — is a very popular option for women. The most common combination is usually a breast augmentation (implants) with or without a breast lift, and a tummy tuck (occasionally with liposuction of the love handles). You can, however, choose almost any combination of procedures and call it a mommy makeover — there are no strict definitions here. For example, you may want to have a rhinoplasty and a tummy tuck, or a breast augmentation and a buttock lift. Just be sure to listen to your plastic surgeon's advice and don't have too many procedures at once.

Before

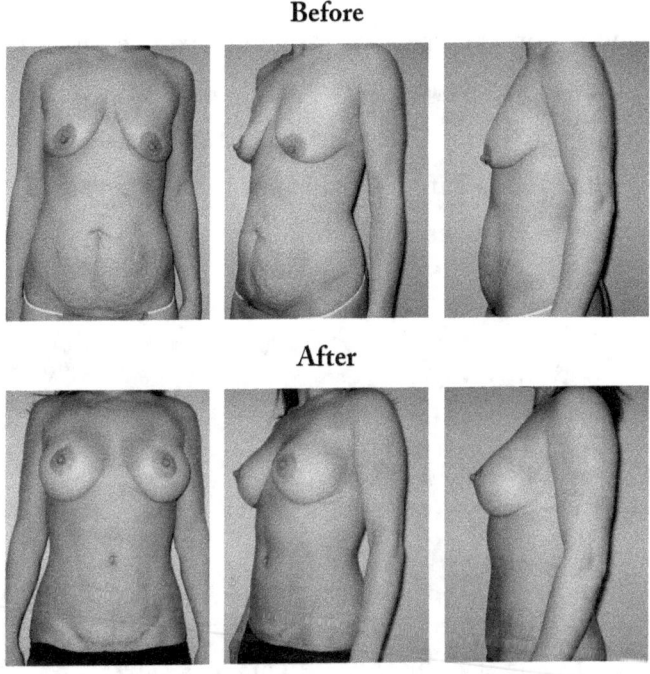

After

32-year-old woman before (top) and after (bottom)
mommy makeover consisting of tummy tuck,
breast lift and 339-cc silicone breast augmentation

There is occasionally temptation on behalf of both patient and surgeon to complete multiple procedures under one anesthesia. Be careful. Safety should be the number one priority for you and your surgeon. You may not be able to accomplish all your cosmetic goals in one day. That's ok. If you need two separate operations on two separate days, sometimes that is the best and safest approach. Too much anesthesia in one day can lead to serious complications. Your surgeon will discuss what is "too much" at the time of your consultation.

Depending on the specific procedures you select, you can expect to take about one to two weeks off to recover. Since a mommy makeover is a very customized surgery, your surgeon will create a safe surgical plan best suited to your unique anatomy and your aesthetic goals.

Ask Dr. Bruno*

Question: How soon after consultation can I have a mommy makeover?

Dr. Bruno: The first priority is that you are in good overall medical health before considering a mommy makeover. You may need to be seen by your primary care physician to have medical clearance prior to surgery. After your consultation, you should meet with the surgeon one more time, perhaps a week later, so that you can ask additional questions that were not addressed at the first visit. You may also want to meet with more than one plastic surgeon to determine which surgeon is right for you.

You could have surgery within days or within weeks/months of your consultation, depending upon the schedule of your surgeon and yourself.

There is no specific time frame between consultation and surgery, but you do need to be in good health (no smoking for two to three weeks, and off all aspirin/ibuprofen products). Please take your time and *don't* rush into an elective procedure.

Question: Can I have multiple procedures in one day?

Dr. Bruno: You may require separate surgeries to complete your goals, but it depends on your health and the length of surgery. Generally speaking, outpatient surgeries should be limited to less than six hours of general anesthesia. This varies, of course, depending on each patient, so a thorough exam is needed to design the best and safest approach.

*Always consult your doctor before having any procedures or treatments

Non- and Minimally Invasive Treatments

Many beauty-enhancing treatments can be done with simple injections or other in-office procedures. You're often in and out within a few hours, you don't have to deal with the side effects of general anesthesia and there's no lengthy recovery time.

Botox and dermal fillers

Botox. When botulinum toxin, or Botox, is administered via injection to the face, it temporarily weakens facial muscles, thereby alleviating wrinkles in the skin. It is quick, simple and relatively inexpensive. You may not see the full effect for a few days, but it typically lasts three to four months.

There's a reason Botox is the number one cosmetic procedure in America: when done properly and at appropriate intervals by a qualified physician, the results are often miraculous. Lines and wrinkles are softened or erased, leaving you with smoother skin. You'll look and feel fresher, without any risk of looking dramatically "different" in a way that will startle anyone. There's also some evidence that Botox treatment can even relieve the muscle tension and nerve strain of migraine headaches.

Some Botox patients experience headaches, nausea, bruising, drooping eyelids and loss of facial expression. Since it is a paralyzing toxin, after all, there are also serious risks if it spreads into other areas of the body. It's important to avoid all aspirin and Motrin-like medications a week before Botox (or any injection), to minimize bruising.

Botox treatments are very quick (usually no more than ten minutes) and have a very short recovery time with no unsightly bruising or swelling. It's convenient and affordable enough to be an occasional supplement to the rest of your beauty regimen.

So remember, Botox weakens muscles. The fillers, however, work differently. Dermal fillers fill in lines. Let's briefly mention some of the common fillers below.

Dermal fillers. A variety of synthetic fillers used to restore lost volume of the face and/or fill in deep lines or wrinkles.

- Hyaluronic acid (known by brand names Restylane,

Juvederm). Typically lasts six to twelve months. Commonly used in the lips, under eyes and nasolabial folds (lines from nose to corner of mouth). Juvederm *Voluma* is similar to Juvederm but is indicated to restore volume to the cheek bone area specifically.

- Calcium hydroxyapatite (Radiesse). Effects may last a year or more, but the material is thick and thus harder to inject. Used mostly for nasolabial folds and/or the cheek area.

- Poly-L-lactic acid (Sculptra). This is useful at restoring lost volume of the midface and cheeks. Typically requires a few injections every two months. Can last one to two years.

There are numerous other products available on the market today and many others in the research and development phase. The products listed above are only a small sampling of some of the more commonly used fillers. Be sure to ask your physician or surgeon which procedure is best for you.

Ask Dr. Bruno*

Question: Is Botox only good for certain face wrinkles and lines, or does it work with all lines and furrows?

Dr. Bruno: Lines on the face caused by excessive facial muscle contraction or movement ("dynamic" lines and wrinkles) respond to Botox treatments. The Botox temporarily weakens the muscle, which relaxes the skin in the area, which creates a smoother look. This is best used for the crow's feet area (sides of the eyes), between the eyes (glabellar area) and the horizontal lines of the foreheads. It can be used in other areas, but should be done conservatively.

Lines caused by aging, such as the nasolabial folds (lines between the nostril and corner of mouth) are not typically treated with Botox and are best treated with fillers (Juvederm, Restylane, Radiesse).

Please consult with a board-certified plastic surgeon for a comprehensive evaluation of your face and of the best treatment options.

Question: What will work for hollow cheeks?

Dr. Bruno: There are several options to restore volume into a hollowed appearing cheek area. Probably the best option is to use your own fat. This will require removing fat from one area (like your abdomen or thigh) and transferring it to your cheek. Not all of the fat will survive, so you may need more than one procedure to get the best results.

Another option is Sculptra, which is polylactic acid and will stimulate the formation of new collagen. This requires a few injection sessions separated by three to six weeks each, and allows for a gradual improvement in the area over time (you will not see the results immediately — the collagen will slowly regenerate). Radiesse is another injectable that can restore volume and stimulate new collagen formation. Both Radiesse and Sculptra can last from one to two years.

*Always consult your doctor before having any procedures or treatments.

Skin treatments

If your skin appears lifeless, discolored, wrinkled, veined or scarred, there are innovative treatments that target each of these conditions. These range from simple skincare programs to deep facial peels; all involve the controlled destruction of skin cells and the encouragement of new skin growth. To determine which ones might be right for you, first you must identify the nature of your skin issues.

Skin discolorations can take a variety of forms: birth marks, freckles, rosacea (redness of the skin), melasma (blotchy areas) and so-called age spots (actually caused by exposure to ultraviolet sun rays). UV rays are also responsible for the fine crêpe paper wrinkles that afflict some people — especially those with fair skin. Acne can leave permanent scarring that detracts from the skin's natural beauty. All of these can be treated with many of the procedures described in this section.

Your skin is continually producing new cells to replace the dead ones on the surface. As you age, that regenerative cycle takes longer, which is why your skin loses tone and color over time. You can help the process along with a doctor-supervised skincare program. This usually begins with an exfoliation or cleansing to remove the dead cells. Then, alpha hydroxyl acids (AHA) and Retin-A may be applied to encourage new growth and thicken the deep skin layers. Bleaching agents, such as hydroquinone, may then be applied to suppress the activities of pigment-producing cells. And finally, moisturizers and sunscreen will protect your newly revitalized skin. All these procedures can be performed by nurses or trained estheticians, but they should always be under the supervision of a qualified dermatologist or plastic surgeon.

Chemical peel. Similar results can be achieved with a superficial chemical peel of glycolic acid, lactic acid or salicylic acid. This procedure is relatively easy and simple, so it has become an attractive add-on service for people in various aspects of the cosmetic industry. Women who have this procedure (usually not more than once a month) may even feel more comfortable going without makeup, since their skin feels smoother and is visibly brighter.

As always, you should *only* have a skin peel from a qualified professional. The procedure may produce mild, temporary burning or itching, and is usually followed with moisturizing cream. Then you can get back to normal activity right away. If you've been using Retin-A, you should stop at least five days before your chemical peel. Of course, all skin treatments should always be followed by good skin maintenance (moisturizers, sunscreen). Some people have this treatment every six to twelve weeks.

Microdermabrasion. This non-invasive procedure involves simply the removal of the top layer of dead skin cells by a machine that acts like a sander. It is often performed before a superficial skin peel to achieve the best results, and you leave with fresher-looking skin that still appears natural. This procedure may be done every four to six weeks.

Laser resurfacing. Lasers are indicated for the treatment of medium to deep lines/wrinkles. Lasers are more expensive than chemical peels, but the results typically last longer. In this process, dead skin is removed layer by layer. It's effective in treating acne scars, wrinkles and discolorations of all types. The procedure is performed by a physician and can take from thirty minutes to two hours. It is an outpatient procedure, but may require sedation or local injections of an anesthetic, depending on the extent of the treatment.

Laser treatments can cause burns, scars or discoloration (the latter of which is usually temporary, but may be permanent). They can also lead to the appearance of cold sores and whiteheads (milia). Lasers can also be used to remove tattoos, spider veins (telangiectasia) and unwanted hair. These processes sometimes require multiple treatments to achieve the desired results.

Fractional laser (Fraxel or non-ablative laser). Offers the results of a deep treatment with the risks of a medium treatment. It does this by treating just twenty percent of the skin each time. It improves fine lines, dynamic wrinkles, large pores, skin texture, discoloration and acne scarring. Because it involves multiple treatments, it avoids the telltale demarcation lines between treated and untreated areas. It can be administered by a nurse with topical anesthesia, with or without oral sedation. Each treatment takes thirty to forty-five minutes, and is not painful. The skin will be red for about a day, and then appear gray and dry for about two weeks. Don't panic! That means it's working. The final result will be baby-smooth skin that shines.

Intense pulsed light (IPL). Improves skin discolorations, fine wrinkles, dull skin, rough skin and large pores. It is also effective in removing unwanted hair. The treatment can be somewhat painful, but there's generally no discomfort afterward, and little recovery time. The primary risk, ironically, is unintended skin coloration, which especially affects dark-skinned people. Some people elect to have two to five treatments, spaced at four- to six-week intervals.

Remember that new laser technologies are constantly being developed, and what may be popular today may be considered obsolete a year or two from now. Consult with an experienced dermatologist or plastic surgeon who is familiar with the latest laser before having any of these procedures.

Ask Dr. Bruno*

Question: I'm forty-one and look good for my age, but would like to be pro-active at this point. What laser treatments for sun damage, fine lines, larger pores and facial redness are best for me to start now?

Dr. Bruno: There are numerous lasers available to treat sun damage and fine lines of aging. Fraxel is an excellent option to rejuvenate your skin and diminish the appearance of fine lines.

In addition to lasers, chemical peels may have a role also in improving the texture of your skin. A good skincare regime should also include a retinol (such as Retin-A) as well as topical vitamin C.

Please consult with a board-certified plastic surgeon or dermatologist to see what treatment or combination of treatments is best for your particular skin type.

*Always consult your doctor before having any procedures or treatments.

Spider veins

Spider veins are the tiny veins that appear on the surface of the skin, not to be confused with varicose veins (which are larger). They can be treated using either of two methods.

- *Sclerotherapy.* The veins are injected with a chemical, causing them to contract and collapse. The process takes about an hour, and usually produces a fifty to ninety percent improvement. Bandages are removed after three to ten days. Multiple sessions may be necessary to achieve the best results.

- *Laser therapy.* This is best for small- to medium-sized spider veins, and for treatments on the face. The laser causes the veins to coagulate and shrink. At first, they'll appear darker and more visible, and then fade over a period of weeks. Like other laser treatments, this one may cause light discoloration (ten to twenty percent of cases), or matting of the veins. Usually three treatments are sufficient, spaced three months apart.

Both of these treatments are permanent, but new spider veins could appear afterward. If varicose veins are present, they must be treated first by a vascular or qualified general surgeon.

That's not all...

The surgeries and procedures described here are some of the most popular treatments sought out by patients. There are, however, many other procedures not listed here that may be right for you. New ones are arriving all the time, and older techniques are constantly being refined. To make it even more confusing, there are also many variations of all these treatments. You may find them represented under other names (e.g., liposuction is also called lipoplasty, liposculpture and lipectomy).

Whatever your cosmetic issue may be, there's almost certainly an effective treatment for it. So let this whet your appetite to discover what's right for you — and then go for it.

We've discussed some of the "What to get?" options for you to consider, but you'll need to plan your next step equally carefully: "Who?"

Chapter 4: Choosing the Right Surgeon

As we've discussed, any licensed physician *can* perform cosmetic procedures; there are currently no state or federal laws preventing them from doing so, or from advertising their services. There are, however, rigorous training programs and professional boards for plastic surgeons, but physicians aren't required to join them. As a result, many physicians have jumped into the field of cosmetic plastic surgery with little training or experience. After all, cosmetic procedures are popular, lucrative and convenient — so practitioners are eager to jump on the bandwagon.

Once you begin thinking about cosmetic surgery, you'll probably start noticing all the advertisements for cosmetic surgeons. They seem to be everywhere! How will you make the best choice?

There is a big difference between a cosmetic surgeon and a plastic surgeon. A plastic surgeon is trained specifically in plastic surgery (both aesthetic and reconstructive). A cosmetic surgeon is a physician trained in a specialty such as dermatology, gynecology or internal medicine, who has one year of training in some cosmetic procedures. We'll elaborate more on this shortly as we discuss "board certification" of doctors.

It goes without saying that any doctor you allow near your body should have a license to practice medicine. The

Federation of State Medical Boards is a good place to confirm the credentials of the surgeon(s) you are considering: http://www.fsmb.org/. This just confirms that the person you are considering is a qualified physician — not a plastic surgeon. You can also check with your state medical board to be sure your doctor is in good standing.

So far, so good. But where do you go from there?

Board certification

While board certification is not strictly legally necessary, it's an excellent way to weed out the less-reputable practitioners. As many as one-third of practicing cosmetic physicians have no board certification whatever! Steer clear of them and do your homework on the rest. Many cosmetic practitioners advertise themselves as "board-certified" without specifying which board they're referring to. Yet there are literally dozens of boards for cosmetic surgeons, some of which are self-appointed, with no endorsement from the larger medical community. To make things worse, the names often sound alike. Differentiating between them can be tricky, but is much easier once you're a little familiar with the terminology.

There are plenty of online resources for locating a plastic surgeon... in fact, perhaps a bit *too* many. A Google search might lead you to numerous websites with the word "cosmetic" or "plastic" in their title. Here a few of the truly important websites you should be familiar with when searching for a plastic surgeon.

The American Board of Plastic Surgery (ABPS) — "the gold standard," as one surgeon calls it — is the most widely recognized board in this field. It is recognized by the American Board of Medical Specialties, an organization that oversees credentialing of legitimate specialty organizations. The ABPS only certifies physicians who have:

- graduated from an accredited medical school.

- completed an accredited residency program.

- been recommended by that program's chairperson.

- passed a written exam.

- submitted a list of the surgeries they've performed.

- passed a two-day oral exam.

- met the ABPS moral and ethical standards.

Physicians who are ABPS-certified can join the American Society of Plastic Surgeons (ASPS). Back in Chapter 1 we learned that the ASPS (founded in 1931) is the oldest professional plastic surgery society in America. They cover reconstructive, aesthetic and hand surgery. You can check the certification status of any plastic surgeon by searching the website: http://www.abplasticsurgery.org/.

On the other hand, there is a board called the American Board of Cosmetic Surgery. This board is not even recognized by the American Board of Medical Specialties (www.ABMS.

org), which oversees all medical specialties in the United States.

Even if a physician claims to be American Board of Cosmetic Surgery-certified, he or she may not necessarily be a specialist in the area of cosmetic surgery. Many internists, emergency room physicians, OB/GYNs, etc., may offer Botox or liposuction as "additional services" to their regular practice. Don't be fooled.

Probably the most prestigious national board related to aesthetic plastic surgery is the American Society for Aesthetic Plastic Surgery (ASAPS). Being a member of the ASAPS means that your surgeon is a legitimate board-certified plastic surgeon and he or she specializes in aesthetic (cosmetic) types of plastic surgery procedures. Check out their website for more information at www.surgery.org.

The point here is to be curious when a physician describes him or herself as "board-certified". Find out what board they have in mind, and then investigate the legitimacy of that board and the doctor's claims. You don't want to go to a gynecologist or internist for a breast augmentation or a tummy tuck, do you?

The internet: your "frenemy" (friend and enemy)

The internet can be a great starting point to begin learning about plastic surgery. There are thousands of websites available — some good, and some not so good. However, be careful not to rely exclusively on the internet for all your information. You will need actual consultations with surgeons to get all your questions answered and to determine if you are even a good surgical candidate.

Online reviews can be invaluable, as they provide unvarnished reports from real consumers. The popular Yelp.com works just as well for finding a plastic surgeon as for finding a good restaurant. Just type in "Plastic Surgery New York" — or whatever your city is — and you'll discover lots of entries. Vitals.com provides consumer reviews for physicians of all types. RealSelf.com provides the same service specifically for those seeking cosmetic services and procedures.

As anyone in any business knows, it's impossible to please everybody. People have bad experiences for all kinds of reasons; they may have begun the day in a bad mood. The service provider may remind them of someone they don't like. The office décor may have turned them off. And such people are usually the quickest to voice their complaints — especially in online forums. So, take such negative reviews with a grain of salt, and weigh them against the positive ones. On the other hand, if a physician has a long string of mostly negative reviews, that's definitely a red flag.

It's also important to note how a professional responds to negative feedback. If a physician's office ignores valid complaints on serious issues, that's a bad sign. If the physician responds defensively, that's just as bad. The professional way to deal with such issues is to display courtesy, empathy and a genuine effort to remedy the problem. A conciliatory attitude in such cases is a sign of strength, not weakness.

Personal referrals are also a great way to find a good plastic surgeon. If you know someone who had a good experience with a particular physician, research the doctor and schedule a consultation — if you feel ready. Don't be afraid to ask your friend lots of questions. "Were the results all that you hoped for? Did the physician explain everything in detail? Did he or she listen to you? Was there anything that disappointed or alarmed you? How did the staff treat you? Was the facility up-to-date and well-maintained?" References from other professionals in the field can be valuable, too. But remember, those people may know the physician only as a colleague, and have no personal experience with his or her work.

When you begin interviewing plastic surgeons, ask if you can see before-and-after pictures, which should be readily available on their website. Look for lots of photos of the procedure you are interested in particular. The more photos a surgeon has of a certain procedure generally indicates he or she performs that procedure with regularity. You might also ask if you could speak to some previous patients to gather even more insight to the surgeon's practice and personality.

There's no substitute for experience

You should be aware that not all plastic surgeons are the same. Just because someone is a board-certified plastic surgeon does not mean they are necessarily proficient in all subspecialties of plastic surgery. Some do a lot more aesthetic (cosmetic) work than others. For example, my practice is a heavy aesthetic practice with very little reconstructive surgery. Breast augmentations, tummy tucks and liposuction are very common procedures that I perform on a daily basis. In contrast, some plastic surgeons specialize in more reconstructive procedures such as breast cancer reconstruction, hand surgery, cleft lips and facial trauma. These plastic surgeons may not be as skilled or comfortable doing tummy tucks and facelifts. By the same token, I no longer do hand surgery or burn reconstruction — I refer those patients to the appropriate specialists.

It's difficult to know exactly which procedures your plastic surgeon is most experienced performing. One way is to simply ask the staff or the surgeon directly. You may ask, for example, "How many breast augmentations do you typically do per month?" I commonly get these types of questions and believe the patient has every right to know that type of information. Hopefully you are consulting with an honest, ethical surgeon who will answer your questions accurately and truthfully. Some plastic surgeons have egos that make them believe they can do any surgery, even if they haven't done that particular procedure in a few years, or even since their residency. This is why it's important to consult with several plastic surgeons (not just one) when making your decision. Again, look for lots of positive reviews and before-

and-after photos online, that will also give you an idea of the types of procedures your surgeon is really good at. If your surgeon doesn't have a lot of tummy tuck photos on his website, it's safe to assume that tummy tucks are not one of his more popular surgeries.

I would also add here that a few non-plastic surgeons are very skilled at certain cosmetic procedures. Some Ear Nose and Throat (ENT) surgeons do beautiful rhinoplasties. Some dermatologists perform fantastic liposuction. In certain cases, these physicians are also ones you may want to look into for specific procedures.

It's important to choose a surgeon who has substantial experience — not just in plastic surgery, but in the *specific* procedure you're considering.

Check the facility, too!

As we've discussed, cosmetic procedures are routinely performed in hospitals, outpatient surgery centers or private physicians' offices. If you have a significant medical history, your surgery may need to be done in a hospital setting with an overnight stay. However, most healthy patients typically undergo cosmetic procedures in an outpatient setting. Regardless of the type of facility you elect to have the procedure performed at, make sure it is an accredited facility.

Along with Medicare, there are three private entities that accredit medical facilities. They assure that facilities meet adequate standards for safety, equipment, office layout and staff. They will also require that a physician have privileges to perform the same procedures at an accredited hospital.

The private accrediting bodies for medical facilities are:

- Accreditation Association for Ambulatory Health Care (AAAHC) — http://www.aaahc.org.

- The Joint Commission (TJC) — http://www.jointcommission.org

- American Association for Accreditation of Ambulatory Surgical Facilities (AAAASF) — http://www.aaaasf.org

Surgeon shopping

After you've done your homework and narrowed down a list of physicians, your next step will probably be an in-person consultation with a few doctors. Some surgeons may offer a free consultation, while others may charge a fee (usually around $150). Be sure to find out when you call to make the appointment whether a fee is required to consult; if it is, ask whether that fee can be applied toward the cost of your surgery (if you end up having one). It's also a good idea to bring a friend, spouse or family member to the consultation, if possible, for support and to ask questions that you may forget to ask.

During this consultation, the physician should give you a thorough explanation of the procedure(s) you're considering. Some may show you videos of the surgery you are interested in. Some may take photographs and use computerized imaging to review your anatomy in greater detail. You can approach this as a question-and-answer session. Of course, you can tackle these questions in any order you like, and often the answer to one will satisfy other questions as well.

Who? "Will the surgeon perform the procedure him or herself? Who else will be present (interns, nurses, anesthesiologist, etc.), and what are their roles? Who will I be seeing after the surgery for follow-up visits?"

What? Information about the procedure itself — "What does it consist of? What are its limitations? What sort of discomfort should I expect during and after the procedure?"

Where? "Will the procedure be done in a hospital, an outpatient surgical facility or the doctor's office?"

When? "What dates are available in my own and the surgeon's schedule to have this procedure done? When do I need to be seen for follow-up? When can I return back to work?"

Why? Ask about the expected results, as well as the potential risks. "Are there alternatives I may want to consider that will achieve the same (or similar) results?" Also consider that you are interviewing the surgeon; the question in your mind should be, "Why should I hire this person to work on my body?"

How? Find out the details about the procedure, recovery and follow-up. "How long does the procedure take? How long until final results are visible?"

Let the surgeon impress you with his or her positive qualities; the focus should be on what can (and cannot) be done for you. Make sure the surgeon is really listening to you, rather than reciting from a rehearsed script. He or she should listen attentively to your questions, and answer thoughtfully, clearly and honestly — even if it's not necessarily the answer you want to hear.

And of course, you'll have some additional questions of your own. You might ask to see before-and-after photos of past patients. Also, be sure to ask whether images of your own procedure will be used in medical publications, website or advertising. You play a crucial role in this consult: now is the time to disclose your full medical history, including allergies, past surgeries, current or past diagnoses that may affect this procedure, any medications you're currently taking, and so on. Don't be afraid or embarrassed — doctors have seen and heard it all, and cannot be shocked. They need to have as complete and honest a picture of your physical and mental health as you are able to provide. If you have any doubts about whether a certain piece of information is relevant, err on the side of telling the doctor and letting him or her decide.

The procedure

Your procedure may take place in a hospital, an outpatient surgery center or a physician's office. As previously mentioned, most young, healthy patients will have their procedure performed at an outpatient surgery center or office-based facility. The majority of patients will be discharged home the same day of the procedure. Some patients may choose to stay overnight at an aftercare facility where nurses can monitor progress for a night or two. This is an option for patients who may not have someone to look after them while at home after surgery.

Those patients with serious medical conditions, such as a cardiac history (for example, a pacemaker), poorly controlled diabetes or high blood pressure, likely should have their procedures done in a hospital setting.

Lights out!

Depending on the surgery, you'll be administered one of three types of anesthesia:

1. *General anesthesia.* This is for most surgeries, including tummy tucks, breast augmentations, large-volume liposuctions and most facial procedures. You are unconscious and your body is motionless, meaning you'll require a breathing tube. You won't remember anything of your surgery once you wake up. Though very rare, complications can include pneumonia, stroke, heart

attack or blood clots in the legs or lungs. This is why an anesthesiologist's one and only job is to monitor the patient's responses and adjust the administration of sedatives as needed to ensure minimal risk.

2. ***IV sedation.*** Also referred to as *twilight sleep* or *monitored anesthesia.* You'll be partially conscious but unaware of what's going on during your surgery. No need for a breathing tube. Some smaller cases of liposuction, for example, can be done under IV sedation.

3. ***Local anesthesia.*** This involves numbing only the area in which the surgery occurs. It's usually appropriate for relatively minor procedures such as lip augmentation or mole removal, and typically lasts one to two hours. Usually the surgeon applies a numbing agent (either topically on the skin or via injection) before injecting the stronger anesthetic.

Recovery

For invasive treatments, remember: no matter how minor, *you have still had a surgical procedure.* This means you'll need to take care of yourself accordingly. Now is not the time to "push through" or "be strong" — your body has experienced trauma from both the anesthetic and the procedure itself, and should not be subjected to the stress of your regular routine (let alone increased activity).

Even if you've had a minimally invasive treatment, the local anesthetic can temporarily affect your thinking and your reflexes. Don't plan to drive yourself home when you leave the facility, and don't try to keep up with your regular daily activities.

Remember, forewarned is forearmed: chances are good that *you will look worse before you look better.* Virtually all plastic surgery causes some swelling and/or bruising. Especially if you've had any kind of facial procedure, plan on spending the first few days looking like you've lost a fight. It can be a shock for a patient who eagerly looks into the mirror to see her new face, only to be confronted with an almost unrecognizable version of herself. This swelling and bruising is actually good news though, since it means your body is working hard to heal itself up (so you can get on with looking fabulous!) This typically peaks within two to three days, and should gradually recede. Your surgeon may recommend you take Arnica or Bromelain before and after surgery, these homeopathic medications can reduce bruising and swelling. Many procedures now use absorbable stitches, which disappear on their own. Otherwise, you'll be asked to revisit the doctor after a few days to have your stitches removed.

Virtually all surgical procedures leave scars, which are permanent. Fortunately, modern techniques can minimize their visibility by clever placement of incisions. These scars usually fade over time, and can take up to one full year to completely lighten in color. Each person heals differently, depending on skin tone, ethnicity, skin thickness and genetics. Exposure to sunlight, especially during the first year, can darken scars. It's best to avoid excessive exposure to sunlight or tanning salons after surgery — or anytime, for that matter. And if you don't already, you should get in the habit of using sunscreen with a sun protection factor (SPF) of at least fifteen, with multi-spectrum protection against UVA *and* UVB light. There are also some very effective silicone gels and tapes that can be applied to incisions after surgery to accelerate the healing process. I routinely have my patients use Biocorneum (silicone gel) and/or Embrace (silicone tape) after surgery as scar therapy.

Some pain and discomfort is common with most surgeries. Your physician will likely prescribe pain medication that will carry you through the recovery period — usually only necessary for a few days. There are also long-lasting local anesthetics, such as Bupivacaine, which can smooth out the period immediately following surgery. There is even a longer-acting version of this medication (called Exparel) that can be used to alleviate pain for up to seventy-two hours after surgery — this is great for tummy tucks!

Your treatment should include follow-up visits, and specific instructions on how to optimize your recovery. You'll need to be diligent to follow these directions regarding work, exercise and other activities.

The risks

All surgery involves risks, and plastic surgery is no exception. The risks vary according to the scope of the procedure, but they are real and serious. You should get familiar with them, and be prepared to face them head-on. Don't think, *"They won't happen to me."* They could! Obviously the major risks (heart attack or death) occur very rarely, and often involve patients who have pre-existing medical conditions. The anesthesia itself (not necessarily the procedure) carries its own risk. Still, you should think carefully and consult with your surgeon and primary care physician before deciding whether to undertake the risks of elective surgery.

The most obvious non-medical risk is that the surgery won't deliver the results you expected. This is not unheard of, and can happen for a number of reasons.

Your initial expectations weren't realistic. You may have envisioned yourself looking like a model or a celebrity after your surgery. But you're still you; no surgery can change that. You may need to work at accepting who you are before attempting to improve your image through surgery. Cosmetic procedures are usually very effective at dealing with certain specific problems, but they're not a cure-all. Just because you show your surgeon a photo of a person you want to look like, doesn't mean you will have that same result.

The physician didn't adequately prepare you. Perhaps the surgeon painted a rosy picture of the likely results. As with such sales pitches, the truth can be disappointing. The best way to avoid that kind of letdown is, of course, to pick a top-quality surgeon who fully explains all aspects of the procedure, including the risks. In any case, you should educate yourself and ask lots of questions beforehand. A physician may show you computer simulations to illustrate the results of a procedure, but these models can't account for all the variables that occur with real, live human beings. You should regard these as simulations only — not precise predictions of what you'll experience.

The procedure didn't go as planned. Of course, no matter how skilled and prepared the physician and staff are, occasionally the results vary from expectations due to technical difficulties with the procedure itself or with a patient's anatomy. Some of your features may appear asymmetrical after surgery. For example, after a breast augmentation you may notice slight asymmetries of your breasts now that they are larger — which were likely present before surgery. If you and your doctor agree that these problems were the result of the surgery and can be corrected with further surgery, you may need to schedule a revision procedure. This is a rare problem for most accepted procedures, but it does occur. (The re-operation rate for breast augmentation is about twenty-five percent within five years. For liposuction, it's five to fifteen percent; for facelifts and eyelid surgery, less than five percent.) You may also experience an early relapse, requiring a repeat surgery sooner than expected.

All these can affect your results and level of satisfaction. You and your surgeon will need to work out, in *advance* (before you have the procedure you're planning), a plan in case you do end up needing revision surgery for some reason. For instance, how much time should you expect to wait before undergoing revision surgery? Will there be an additional charge, and if so, who will pay for it?

There are also other risks that accompany surgery. These include:

- Infection (addressed with antibiotics).

- Pain (can be alleviated with long-lasting local anesthetics such as Bupivacaine).

- Hematoma (a mass of clotted blood in the area of the surgery).

- Seroma (a collection of fluid in the area of the surgery).

- Skin necrosis (dead skin which must be surgically removed).

- Numbness /tingling (usually temporary — but not always).

- Paralysis or weakness (caused by damage to nerves).

There are other risks associated with specific procedures, which you should explore fully with your physician before undergoing any treatment. Please take the time to review the informed consent and ask questions prior to agreeing to any elective procedure.

The long term

Some procedures, such as nose surgery and chin implants, are permanent. Others, such as a facelift or breast lift, last for a finite period of time and may need to be repeated to maintain the effects. You should be very clear about the longevity of any procedure you undertake. The final results of your procedure may not be evident for weeks, months or even years (rhinoplasty, for example, often requires about one year for the nose to settle into its final shape). Before having any procedure, discuss the specific time frame of recovery with your surgeon in detail.

Chapter 5: Go for It!

You're now pretty well-acquainted with the world of plastic surgery. You have an idea of what's available, and have probably zeroed in on the procedure(s) that interest you. Now it's time to develop a plan. If that seems intimidating, it'll be easier if you break it down into small, workable steps.

1. Decide if you're ready.

You've come this far, but you haven't committed to anything yet. That's good — you're bringing your intelligence and forethought to the process.

Self questions:

- Is this something I really want to do? Why?

- Do I want to do it now? If not, when?

- Are my expectations realistic?

- Am I prepared for the risks?

- Am I in a position to pay for it or finance it right now?

- Will I really commit to the necessary recovery and follow-up?

If the answer to any of these is *no*, don't sweat it. You may be ready in the future. Feel free to put it aside for now, think things over, and then pick it up again later. Remember, this is elective surgery, so there's no reason to rush into anything.

If all your answers are *yes*, fasten your seatbelt and read on.

2. Do your homework.

You already know something about the procedures you're considering. But make it your goal to become even better informed. The lists here can help you organize your research and determine the kinds of questions to ask, as well as keep track of the (sometimes different) answers you may get.

Procedure questions:

- What will happen during this procedure?

- What specific results are intended?

- What are the risks (physical, emotional, financial)?

- Where will the procedure be performed, and why?

- Is the facility accredited? By whom?

- How long does this procedure typically take?

- How much pain/discomfort is typical, and how long does it last?

- What kind of anesthetic will be used during the procedure?

- Can the doctor administer a long-lasting local anesthetic as well?

- What should I be sure to do — or NOT to do — during recovery?

- How long will it take for final results to be evident?

- What is the likelihood of revision surgery?

- When will we know if revision surgery becomes necessary for me, and if so, when will we be able to do it and what costs will it entail?

3. Choose the best surgeon you can afford.

If ever there was a field where the saying, "You get what you pay for," holds true, it's this one. Price doesn't tell you everything, but it can be an indicator of quality. If a surgeon is at the bottom of the price scale, he or she may be just beginning a practice, or trying to overcome a bad reputation. Either way, it's good to look elsewhere. On the other hand, exorbitant fees don't guarantee quality. Plastic surgery in this country has become somewhat of a commodity to some people. Patients may think that anyone can do a breast augmentation, so why not go for the cheapest price — the results are all the same in their eyes. This could not be further from the truth. Be very careful and only use cost as one small factor when making your decision on which surgeon to choose. Also, if you are considering having surgery outside of the United States, be very careful, because if you develop a complication you will likely not have immediate access to your surgeon for post-operative care. International facilities and surgeons are not held to the same strict standards as they are here.

Cost questions:

- What is the estimated TOTAL cost of this procedure, including surgeon's fee, anesthesia, facility, etc.?

- What materials need to be purchased (garments or bras)? Will the doctor provide them or do I need to purchase them myself?

- What additional fees (medications or lab work) should I know about?

You may be able to find answers to some of these questions through your online research, but it's always a good idea to discuss them with the doctor as well.

Don't be shy about asking. It's your life. Make sure you're working with someone who truly cares about you and understands your needs. Also, it's your money, so make sure it's well spent. Select a pool of prospective surgeons based on experience, qualifications and good reviews. Then interview the best ones you can afford.

Doctor questions:

- How long have you been practicing?

- How many times have you performed this specific procedure?

- What board certifications do you have?

- At what hospital(s) do you have privileges?

- What problems have you encountered in performing this procedure?

- How satisfied have your patients been overall?

4. Set realistic expectations.

We're all prone to wishful thinking. But when you're about to spend lots of money and possibly alter your body forever, it's time to be clear-headed. Plastic surgery will change your body — not your life. Listen to the descriptions of what you're likely to experience, and take them seriously. Don't embellish them. You'll probably be delighted with your results. But you'll still be you. Be happy with that.

5. Make the call.

You've done everything you can to make your dream happen… except to book the appointment. It's natural to get cold feet at this point. But if you've decided that you really are ready, take a deep breath, and schedule your procedure. Once you have a date set, your surgeon's office will likely schedule a "pre-op" visit, where you can meet with the surgeon again, a week or so before surgery, to ask more questions and review pre-operative instructions.

6. Prepare for the procedure.

You've got some planning to do. You'll probably need to take time off from work. And don't skimp on the recovery period; take at least as much time as the physician recommends. Also, have you arranged for a ride to and from the facility? If you've had any kind of sedation, you won't be in any shape to drive. Do you have someone to take care of your kids, or your pets? Do you need to fill prescriptions? Where/when do you go to get your blood work done? Your surgeon's patient care coordinator will be able to assist you with answering all of these questions.

As you see, there's a lot to think about. Here's a partial planning checklist. But you may want to add to it, to personalize it for yourself.

Preparation questions:

- Have I arranged for time off work (both for the procedure and recovery)?

- If I have obligations to family, are they aware that I'm having this procedure, and do they know what to expect during my recovery? If necessary, do I have someone to help me care for my children?

- Do I have someone to do errands and household activities for me? Do I need someone to help prepare meals for me?

- If I won't be able to care for my pets — feeding, walking, grooming, etc. — while I recover, is there someone else to do it?

- Do I have a ride to and from the facility where my procedure will be done? (Remember that you should not drive if you've had any anesthesia.)

- If I need any special garments or bras, will my surgeon provide them for me?

- Will I be able to fill my prescription for pain medication right away? Or, have I arranged for someone else to do it? Also, am I prepared for the possible side effects of my pain medication?

7. Follow-up.

Most patients are seen the day after surgery back at their doctor's office for a post-operative visit. Be sure you have someone to drive you to this appointment. You will likely then be seen about one week later to remove any stitches or drains, if necessary. You may be able to drive yourself to the one-week follow-up visit, if you are no longer taking your pain medications. After that, you will likely be seen about a month later, and then three or four months after that, depending on your surgeon's protocol and how you are progressing.

Be sure to follow your surgeon's post-operative instructions carefully. You will be informed when you can return to your usual activities and exercise program. Don't be too eager to return to strenuous activity as you may injure yourself or harm your result.

From here on, it's up to you. Remember: you're in control of your choices. Your new and improved self could be just around the corner. Here's to great results and a bright future!

About the Author

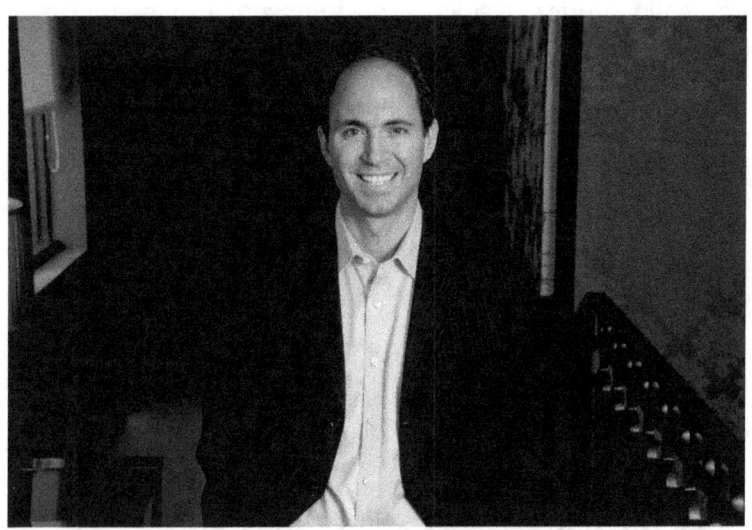

William Bruno, MD

Originally from the East Coast, William Bruno knew from a young age that he wanted to be a physician. When he was just four years old, he was diagnosed with juvenile rheumatoid arthritis, and spent a lot of time visiting doctors and seeing medical specialists. By the time he was seven, William had made a full recovery and his career path in medicine was set.

Certification and Training

Dr. Bruno earned his medical degree from Hahnemann University School of Medicine in Pennsylvania, after completing his premedical studies at Washington University in Saint Louis. He then embarked on his advanced training — which included a surgical internship at Stanford University, the chief surgical residency post at Saint Louis University Medical Center, sub-specialization in microsurgery at Eastern Virginia Medical Center and formal plastic surgery training at Duke University Medical Center, where he practiced cosmetic and reconstructive surgery. Dr. Bruno is board-certified by the American Board of Plastic Surgery (ABPS) and is an active member of the American Society of Plastic Surgeons (ASPS) and the American Society for Aesthetic Plastic Surgery (ASAPS).

In his own words...

Why Become a Plastic Surgeon?

I wanted to do plastic surgery as my specialty for the longest time because I really liked the creativity and artistry of it, versus general surgery. With plastic surgery you're working on men and women — and on all parts of the body. It's challenging and always evolving — there's more than one way to approach a problem. As a child, I used to draw and sketch a lot. Now the work that I'm doing with my patients is again really creative. I try not to impose too much of my aesthetic on patients — I really want to make them happy and am careful to listen to what their goals are.

Why Beverly Hills?

Coming from the East Coast, I'm not that crazy about freezing cold winters. Honestly, I wanted to move to a city that was warm, so for me, the decision came down to Los Angeles or Miami. I had some friends who were working in Hollywood and, obviously, from a plastic surgery perspective, having a Beverly Hills-based practice is the pinnacle for our profession. I love it here. Many of our patients are local, and live in Beverly Hills or West Hollywood, but we also get a number of patients who fly in from all over the world.

What Makes William Bruno Plastic Surgery Different?

First of all, we are a highly specialized boutique practice. About ninety-nine percent of my practice focuses on aesthetic plastic surgery — primarily of the breast, body and buttocks. By combining medicine and artistry, we pride ourselves on providing our patients with attractive, natural-looking results, and putting their safety and comfort first. Second, because we are a small, highly specialized team, it means our patients have direct access to me — from the initial consult all the way through to post-recovery. When they call to speak to me, they don't have to jump through hoops before they get put through. Patients even have my mobile phone number after surgery for questions. I think that having the individualized attention of your surgeon is essential.

What a New Patient Can Expect
from an Initial Consult?

An initial consult to me is always a discovery session — both for me and for the patient. I usually do a lot of listening during these appointments, so that I can really understand what a patient's goals are and what's troubling them. Then I'll discuss some options for the patient and we move into the education aspects of the consult — for example, if a patient is considering a breast augmentation, we'll discuss the differences in silicone versus saline implants and I'll explain the surgical procedure with visual aids. Then, using our TouchMD computer software, we'll take a few photos and review the patient's anatomy and surgical plan. That way they can go home, discuss their options with their family, think about what we discussed and make their own decision. If a patient is considering having a tummy tuck or Brazilian buttock lift, for example, the process is very similar. I think it's critical to take photos and review them with each patient during a consultation. Asymmetries can be pointed out and realistic goals can be set. It's really important during an initial consultation that the patient gets answers to all their questions. I recommend that patients visit with a few plastic surgeons before making their decision. If I'm the first one, I feel they should visit at least one other plastic surgeon for an initial consultation. That way they have multiple perspectives and can make the best decision for themselves.

About His Practice

Dr. Bruno's practice is located on Sunset Boulevard in West Hollywood, California, overlooking the Sunset Strip. He has been in private practice in the Beverly Hills/West Hollywood area since 2004. He performs over 300 surgical procedures a year, in addition to numerous non-surgical injectable procedures. Some of the most common surgeries Dr. Bruno performs are breast augmentations, breast lifts, tummy tucks, liposuction, Brazilian buttock lifts and "mommy makeovers".

All procedures are performed in an accredited surgical center, and patients receive attentive care throughout the process, from personal consultations with Dr. Bruno, to pre-operative medical examinations, to surgery and recovery. Their goal is to *exceed* your expectations for both your surgical outcome and your experience with their practice.

Contact **William Bruno Plastic Surgery** *to learn more. Visit http://www.williambrunomd.com/ or call (310) 461-3855.*

Patient Reviews

Here are a few taken directly from RealSelf.com — visit their website to see more reviews, read Dr. Bruno's answers to questions and much more.

"After working in the field of plastic surgery for many years, I chose Dr. Bruno to do my breast augmentation and liposuction because he was the surgeon that consistently had excellent surgical outcomes with minimal discomfort. All the employees that worked with him in the operating room and in the office also chose him as their surgeon because they knew he was honest, ethical, safe and professional. I will continue to send my friends and family to him for many years to come."

"At first I was very nervous, it was my first procedure but DR Bruno explained the procedure to me the befores the afters and the right nows and it eased me big time. I am beyond satisfied with the results… so many compliments and best part of it all that although very noticeably different it looks so natural. He is seriously awesome. The after post-op appts have made it a lot more comforting as well as he sees me and makes sure everything is as should."

"After years of thorough consideration and research, I opted for aesthetic surgery with Dr. B. I have been exposed to the work of various physicians and no other work, came close to Dr. B's meticulous expertise, professional demeanor and above all exquisite results. I highly recommend Dr. B. He is genuinely compassionate to the needs of his patients. I confirm this firsthand, He is devout to your safety, wellbeing and dedicated to help you achieve your realistic aesthetic goals. Dr. B gave me the peace of mind I needed to make my informed decision. I felt safe in his hands, pre-surgery, throughout the procedure and post recovery. After meeting Dr. B, I could not see myself going through this process elsewhere. I am forever grateful for Dr. B, the physician that made all of the difference."

"Dr. Bruno is amazing! He listens to you, and is very realistic :)! His work is done very well, he can actually give you a naturally big looking butt! His work is so great compared to all the doctors I've researched. He will give you a round booty! No square shapes, very neat! I couldn't be happier with picking him as my doctor. Absolutely NO regrets, I know it's only day 3 but I'm still very happy. If you're in LA, pick him! He uses "pure fat" I had minimal bruising! Thank you Dr. Bruno, my vision of a butt I've wanted for many years has come to life! Thank you!!"

"I've been going to Dr. Bruno over the last few years for botox and juvederm and he is hands down the best that I've been to for these procedures and at 40, I've been to quite a few! The difference with him, is that he has an incredible eye for knowing exactly where and how much to inject so that the lines are removed and volume is added in all the right places, yet I don't look all botox and juvied out like so many other women. No one ever guesses my age. I look NATURALLY younger, and my close girlfriends who do botox and fillers can attest to this, as many have commented that they can usually tell when someone has this work done, but can't tell on me; that I just look naturally younger and wrinkle-free. Needless to say, I've converted many others over to him and they're all obsessed with him now too. Some have now gotten lasers and even plastic surgery and all I can say is, we love him — he does beautiful work and we're all ecstatic that we have a great resource to go to for our anti-aging needs over the years to come. Yay for that."

www.ingramcontent.com/pod-product-compliance
Lightning Source LLC
Chambersburg PA
CBHW071821200526
45169CB00018B/577